Clear-Cutting Disease Control

Rodrick Wallace · Luis Fernando Chaves
Luke R. Bergmann · Constância Ayres
Lenny Hogerwerf · Richard Kock
Robert G. Wallace

Clear-Cutting Disease Control

Capital-Led Deforestation, Public Health Austerity, and Vector-Borne Infection

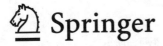 Springer

Rodrick Wallace
New York State Psychiatric Institute
Columbia University
New York, NY, USA

Luke R. Bergmann
Department of Geography
University of Washington
Seattle, WA, USA

Lenny Hogerwerf
Centre for Infectious Disease Control
National Institute for Public Health
and the Environment
Bilthoven, The Netherlands

Robert G. Wallace
Institute for Global Studies
University of Minnesota
Minneapolis, MN, USA

Luis Fernando Chaves
Programa de Investigación en Enfermedades
Tropicales
Universidad Nacional
Heredia, Costa Rica

Constância Ayres
Instituto Oswaldo Cruz
Funação Oswaldo Cruz
Rio de Janeiro, Brazil

Richard Kock
Pathobiology and Population Sciences
The Royal Veterinary College
Hatfield, UK

ISBN 978-3-030-10277-7   ISBN 978-3-319-72850-6 (eBook)
https://doi.org/10.1007/978-3-319-72850-6

Printed on acid-free paper

This Springer imprint is published by Springer Nature
The registered company is Springer International Publishing AG
The registered company address is: Gewerbestrasse 11, 6330 Cham, Switzerland

Preface

The vector-borne flavivirus Zika joins among other infections avian influenza, Ebola, and yellow fever as recent public health crises of regional scale threatening pandemicity. A growing literature situates the origins of many of these emergent outbreaks in changes in land use spearheaded by neoliberal agricultural production as well as mining, logging, and other modes of multinational development. Ecosystems in which "wild" viruses are in part controlled by environmental stochasticity are being drastically streamlined by capital led deforestation and, at the other end of periurban development, by deficits in public health and environmental sanitation.

While many sylvatic pathogens are dying out with their host species as a result, a subset of infections that once burned out relatively quickly in the forest, if only by an irregular rate of host encounter, are now propagating across susceptible human populations whose vulnerability to infection is often exacerbated in urban environments. The resulting outbreaks are characterized by greater extent, duration, and momentum.

In this monograph, we explore an associated bifurcation in the state space of vector-borne outbreaks. The stabilizing effect of environmental "noise" on such infections can be lost in deforestation and, at the other geographic terminus, urban austerity. But by sufficient noise added to a two-dimensional pathogen-vector system of Itô stochastic differential equations, it appears a pathogen population can also become suddenly destabilized, with sequentially rising peaks in infection a characteristic outcome. The results imply that policy-determined noise can as much promote as retard pathogen transmission.

We propose the two impacts together explain the explosive spread of recent vector-borne infections. Whereas stripping out forest for monoculture production or divesting from sanitation removes ecological curbs on vector-borne diseases, the noise associated with socially driven spatial shifts in vector dynamics can propel infection spikes. More generally, an agribusiness-led "neoliberal frontier" spreading across much of the global south, in combination with structural adjustment programs in public health, at one and the same time appears to remove the ecosystemic brake on vector-borne infections and accelerate their subsequent transmission.

We review the implications of such a socially driven bifurcation for intervention and modeling alike. In contrast to what much of the disease literature presumes, in the context of the modern nation state, infectious diseases cannot be described by interacting populations of host, vector, and pathogen alone. We follow up with a series of control theory models that explicitly address the interactions between public health bureaucracies and the pathogens they aim to control.

New York, NY, USA   Rodrick Wallace
Heredia, Costa Rica   Luis Fernando Chaves
Seattle, WA, USA   Luke R. Bergmann
Rio de Janeiro, Brazil   Constância Ayres
Bilthoven, The Netherlands   Lenny Hogerwerf
Hatfield, UK   Richard Kock
Minneapolis, MN, USA   Robert G. Wallace

Contents

About the Authors

Constância Ayres is the vice-director of Fiocruz in Recife and research coordinator of the Oswaldo Cruz Foundation. She holds a PhD in cellular and molecular biology from the Oswaldo Cruz Foundation and a postdoctoral fellowship from the Liverpool School of Tropical Medicine. She has experience in genetics, with emphasis on the genetics of insect populations, working mainly with *Aedes aegypti*, *Culex quinquefasciatus*, and *Anopheles* spp.

Luke R. Bergmann is an assistant professor in the Department of Geography at the University of Washington, USA. His research explores how globalization affects human-environment relations through several thematic focuses. These include changes in the evolution and spread of pathogens, as well as studies of shifting sociospatial relationships between carbon, land use, capital, and consumption.

Luis Fernando Chaves is a visiting researcher at the Programa de Investigación en Enfermedades Tropicales (PIET), Universidad Nacional, Heredia, Costa Rica, and a consultant at the Instituto Conmemorativo Gorgas De Estudios de la Salud, Ciudad de Panamá, Panamá. He is a specialist in medical entomology, mathematical modeling, and vector-borne disease ecology. His focus is on modeling the ecology and control of vectors and the diseases they transmit, with emphasis on leishmaniasis, malaria, and Chagas disease under climate change. Central to his work is the mathematical analysis of natural processes and simulations of simple to complex scenarios that together formally articulate interactions of organisms and the environment. His work spans the study of malaria resurgence in East Africa to the effect of climate cycles of cutaneous leishmaniasis and the effect of temperature and precipitation on West Nile infection in Illinois.

Lenny Hogerwerf is an epidemiologist and disease ecologist at the Centre for Infectious Disease Control (CIb) of the National Institute for Public Health and the Environment (RIVM) of the Netherlands. She obtained her PhD on the epidemiology of Q fever in dairy goat herds in the Netherlands at the Department of Farm Animal Health of the Faculty of Veterinary Medicine of Utrecht University. She has developed a variety of ecological models for explaining the dynamics of HPAI H5N1 and disease landscapes more generally. She has consulted for the Food and Agriculture Organization and Vétérinaires Sans Frontières Belgium.

Richard Kock is a wildlife veterinarian, researcher, and conservationist. He is the chair in wildlife health and emerging diseases at the Pathobiology and Population Sciences Department at the Royal Veterinary College in Hatfield, UK. For over three decades, he has participated in a variety of research and management efforts in epizoology, wildlife health, and conservation in countries around the world, including across sub-Saharan Africa. His most recent projects include the eradication of rinderpest, the characterization of the emergence of virulent *Pasteurella* in saiga antelopes, and efforts to control foot-and-mouth disease and equine piroplasmosis in wild populations in a context of increasing agricultural intensification.

Robert G. Wallace is a public health phylogeographer presently visiting the University of Minnesota's Institute for Global Studies. His research has addressed the evolution and spread of influenza, the agroeconomics of Ebola, the social geography of HIV/AIDS in New York City, the emergence of Kaposi's sarcoma herpesvirus out of Ugandan prehistory, and the evolution of infection life history in response to retrovirals. Wallace is coauthor of *Neoliberal Ebola: Modeling Disease Emergence from Finance to Forest and Farm* (Springer) and *Farming Human Pathogens: Ecological Resilience and Evolutionary Process* (Springer). He has been consulted by the Food and Agriculture Organization of the United Nations and the Centers for Disease Control and Prevention, USA.

Rodrick Wallace is a research scientist in the Division of Epidemiology of the New York State Psychiatric Institute at Columbia University. He received an undergraduate degree in mathematics and a PhD in physics from Columbia University, worked a decade as a public interest lobbyist, and is a past recipient of an Investigator Award in Health Policy Research from the Robert Wood Johnson Foundation. He is the author of numerous books and papers relating to public health and public order.

Chapter 1
The Social Context of the Emergence of Vector-Borne Diseases

Check for
updates

1.1 Introduction

The Brazilian strain of Zika virus (ZIKV-BR) is one of several recently emergent or reemergent vector-borne human infections, pathogens transmitted by the bite of an infected arthropod species (Dick et al. 1952; Kindhauser et al. 2016; Wilder-Smith et al. 2017). The new Zika strain is transmitted, as are other major arboviruses, by *Aedes* spp. mosquitoes, with some debate as to whether other mosquito genera can transmit the virus (Ayres 2016; Fernandes et al. 2016; Evans et al. 2017; Hunter 2017). Its progenitor appears to have originated in Senegal and Côte d'Ivoire before spreading across Asia and more recently, and explosively, South and Central America (Musso 2015; Shen et al. 2016; Faria et al. 2017). Suitable New World niches extend beyond areas struck so far (Messina et al. 2016; Attaway et al. 2017) (Fig. 1.1).

Although Messina et al. (2016) focus primarily on the range of the primary Zika vector – *Aedes aegypti* – as determining the possible extent of the epidemic, the team comments in passing:

> How the ongoing epidemic unfolds in terms of case numbers (or incidence) will depend on a range of other factors such as local transmission dynamics, herd immunity, patterns of contact among mosquitoes and infectious and susceptible humans...and mosquito-to-human ratios as recently shown for dengue...and chikungunya....

Here, we specifically focus on the "range of other factors" that drive vector-borne disease, factors that extend well beyond the list, largely around vectorial capacity, that Messina et al. present. These additional factors are largely matters of socioeconomic structure and public policy, framing the living conditions of human and vector populations (Levins et al. 1994; Lindsay and Birley 2004; Chaves and

© Springer International Publishing AG 2018
R. Wallace et al., *Clear-Cutting Disease Control*,
https://doi.org/10.1007/978-3-319-72850-6_1

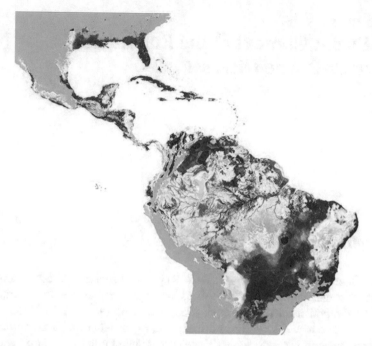

Fig. 1.1 Projected niche susceptibility to the spread of Zika via the *Aedes* mosquito vector in the New World. Gray is zero, bright red high (adapted from Messina et al. 2016)

Koenraadt 2010; Samy et al. 2016; Tusting et al. 2016; Chitunhu and Musenge 2016; Oviedo-Pastrana et al. 2017; Zellweger et al. 2017).

Context may extend beyond immediate anthropogenic conditions, among them access to water and environmental sanitation. Structural One Health, a new field, examines the impacts global circuits of capital and other foundational contexts, including deep cultural histories, have upon regional agroeconomics and associated disease dynamics across species (Wallace et al. 2015; Degeling et al. 2015; Jones et al. 2017; Kingsley and Taylor 2017; Dzingirai et al. 2017). In one such line of research, Wallace and Wallace (2016) modeled the mechanisms by which neoliberal development promoted the emergence of the Ebola Makona strain that infected up to 35,000 West Africans during 2013–2015.

Neoliberalism is a program of political economy aimed at globalizing economic liberalism, promoting free trade, and applying strong state techno-management to protecting private property and deregulating or rather re-regulating corporate-led economic markets (Harvey 2005; Mirowski 2009; Centeno and Cohen 2012; Ganti 2014). It is the latest iteration of capitalism as an actively constructed system of social reproduction, as a totalizing episteme opposed to alternatives, organized over geographic centers and peripheries within and across countries around the globe (Harvey 1982/2006; Mirowski 2009). Neoliberal doctrine impacts local landscapes and functional ecosystems alike, with decisive effect upon the fortunes of infectious disease (Maye et al. 2012; Wallace and Kock 2012; Jones et al. 2013; Maye et al. 2014; Schrecker and Bambra 2015; Wallace and Wallace 2016).

Although the Ebola epidemic Wallace and Wallace (2016) modeled originated in a reservoir species in West Africa – presumably displaced fruit or insectivore bat populations – it rapidly became human-transmissible, permitting direct mathematical modeling, at least in the initial stage. Most simply for such an outbreak, one can write a deterministic "exploding" equation as

$$dX / dt = \alpha X(t) \tag{1.1}$$

at time t where, in the early stages, X is the infected population and α is a positive real number so that $X(t)$ increases exponentially in time:

$$X(t) = X_0 \exp[\alpha t] \tag{1.2}$$

Wallace and Wallace (2016) report the solution unlikely under sufficiently stochastic circumstances. An Itô stochastic differential equation presents

$$dX_t = \alpha X_t dt + \sigma X_t dW_t \tag{1.3}$$

The second term represents volatility in the white "noise" dW_t, a random noise signal with equal power within a fixed bandwidth at any center of frequency, whose influence here is indexed by the parameter σ.

Applying the Itô Chain Rule, a stochastic version of computing the derivative of the composition of two or more functions, to log[X] produces the relation

$$d\log[X_t] = \left(\alpha - \frac{\sigma^2}{2}\right)dt + \sigma dW_t \tag{1.4}$$

where $-\sigma^2/2$ is the "Itô correction factor." Heuristically, given enough environmental noise, i.e., $\sigma^2/2 > \alpha$, by Jensen's inequality for a concave function (Cover and Thomas 2006), this gives a lower limit for $\log[E(X_t)] \geq E(\log[X_t]) \rightarrow a < 0$. That is, any outbreak must eventually be driven to extinction.

More generally, for non-Brownian "colored" noise, with skewed spectral densities of a variety of distributions, if Eq. (1.3) can be expressed as

$$dX_t = X_t dY_t \tag{1.5}$$

where Y_t is a stochastic process in some complicated noise process dB_t, then the Doléans-Dade exponential (Protter 1990), the solution of a class of stochastic differential equations defined by a semimartingale of bounded variation, can be written as

$$E(X)_t \propto \exp\left(Y_t - \frac{1}{2}[Y_t,Y_t]\right)$$

$$(1.6)$$

$[Y_t, Y_t]$ is the quadratic variation of Y_t that, since B_t is not Brownian white noise, need not be simply proportional to time (Protter 1990). Then, again heuristically, by the Mean Value Theorem, if

$$\frac{1}{2}d[Y_t,Y_t]/dt > dY_t/dt \qquad\qquad (1.7)$$

the exponential converges in probability to zero.

Using similar methods, Dalal et al. (2007) found that the introduction of stochastic noise can change the basic reproductive number of a disease and can stabilize an otherwise unstable system. Gray et al. (2011) take an analogous approach to the susceptible-infected-susceptible epidemic. Yang and Mao (2013) found that for a susceptible-exposed-infected-recovered epidemic model, when perturbations are sufficiently large, the exposed and infective components decay exponentially to zero, while the susceptible components converge weakly to a class of explicit stationary distributions regardless of the magnitude of the reproductive number.

With some modification, we can apply the approach to vector-borne disease. Since human-to-human transmission is (relatively) rare for such diseases, mathematical description, following the Ross-Macdonald model of vector-borne infection (Bailey 1975, 1982), requires tracking interactions across multiple species at different time scales. Our particular concern will be the shift from a low deterministic endemic state to high-level stochastic outbreaks.

The transmission system has a minimal two-dimensional setting at the initial state: two interacting populations described by two linked equations. As in the one-dimensional Ebola system discussed above, the right kind of noise can still drive an endemic level in such a system to zero, consonant with, but different from, the Doléans-Dade exponential. On the other hand, the wrong kind of noise can now trigger an explosion of infections.

The ecological processes associated with such definitional environmental noise arise from multiple sources and are almost entirely framed by matters of public policy. For instance, rain repeatedly creates the right conditions for oviposition, but by a nexus of unrelated events that a model's noise spectra can capture, predation and canopy cover, the latter influencing rainfall and sun radiation, can check tree-hole mosquito population growth (Miyagi and Toma 1980; Mogi and Sota 1996; Chaves 2017). When such natural control mechanisms are stripped out by the landscape changes imposed by globalized commodity production, previously marginalized vectors, and their pathogens, are suddenly sprung free from the repeated interruptions of the everyday ecology of the forest.

In contrast, environmental noise (of a variety of empirically discoverable colors) appears inherent to other modes of social development, including traditional, artisanal, and conservation agroecologies that are heavily mosaicked in space, time, kinds of crops and livestock, ecosystemic function, and genetic variability (e.g., Kock 2010; Rosales-Castillo et al. 2011; Wang et al. 2011; Le Flohic et al. 2013; Maas et al. 2016). Ending such systems appears to come at grave epidemiological cost few analyses have formally modeled.

Wallace and Wallace (2016) asserted a shift out of regional agroforestry to capital-led trajectories of neoliberal agriculture, mining, and logging – all highly dependent on global circuits of capital and the expectations of international financial centers as far flung as New York, London, and Hong Kong – imposed a new, epidemiologically critical spatial pattern upon West Africa's forest ecologies. Marginal strains of regional Ebola undertook a punctuated domain shift in spillover and subsequent human transmission. The stripped landscapes replaced traditional if also historically contingent agroecological practices with increasingly uniform ecosystemic "smoothing" that among its many effects increased the interface between reservoir bat species and, by structural adjustment's impacts on public health, elongated chains of human susceptibles. So while at the start of the outbreak in West Africa the virus itself appeared little different from its predecessors at the genetic, molecular, and clinical levels, the outbreak, spreading upon a different transmission background, proved unprecedented in its extent, duration, and momentum.

We propose the emergence (or reemergence) of a wide variety of vector-borne pathogens is framed by a similar – albeit taxa- and place-specific – context.

1.2   The Social Determinants of Vector-Borne Disease

A comprehensive review by Mandal et al. (2011) shows the essential role of social, economic, and political conditions for at least one vector-borne disease, malaria, is well known, if also little studied by way of the traditional systems of simultaneous equations:

> It is now fairly evident that "*as a general rule of thumb, where malaria prospers most, human societies have prospered least*"... Poverty is largely concentrated in the tropical and subtropical zones, and that is where most malaria transmission is observed. The extent of the correlation suggests that malaria and poverty are intimately related. In most endemic areas of malaria, changes in social and economic conditions are considered to be far more important than temperature shift... The economic and social burdens from factors such as fertility, population growth, premature mortality, misdiagnosis, inflicted by the disease have been studied by many authors... Given the nature of the factors, most investigations are case studies, and there are only a few differential equation based models that incorporate socioeconomic structure (e.g., Yang and Ferreira 2000).

About the deficiencies in most such models, focused entirely on the internal interactions between pathogen, host, and vector populations, Bailey (1982) remarks:

> Perhaps none will fully understand the behaviour of the whole system as it operates within the economic, social and political constraints of a given society. This may explain some of the difficulties of predicting with sufficient accuracy the likely consequences of any chosen strategy of intervention. And if one cannot predict the consequences of a given strategy, one had no rational basis for choosing between the available alternatives.

Here we will formally address the influence of some of the key economic, social, and political constraints missing in previous models. To do so, following Finley-Brook (2007), we need to first summarize the development strategies to which the post-WWII global south has been subjected:

The oppressed and poor are supposed to gain freedom through [the neoliberal] market, but neoliberal approaches are not designed to address the particular attributes and needs of native groups... In Latin America many indigenous areas are communally owned. Market-oriented ventures in communal areas that start off as communal risk strengthening local elite, increasing economic and social inequity, or disrupting collective structures... Insensitive to local practices, donors often require the purchase of outside inputs like agricultural machinery, trucks, and cattle. As they attempt to diffuse desire for foreign goods and a culture of consumption, aid agencies spur rapid and often destabilizing technological shifts in rural areas.

Huddell (2010) describes these circumstances as they are instantiated in Brazil:

Neoliberal reforms, which reduced subsidies and government intervention as well as liberalized markets, had complex repercussions for Brazil's agricultural sector. The impact on Brazil's coffee market is illustrative... Market competitiveness favored capital-intensive landowners and foreign interests, and thus marginalized small rural farmers. Exposing the small-scale farmers of Brazil to the world economy, at a time when world coffee prices fell dramatically low, forced them out of the market. The new policies also encouraged mass production, expansion of farmland, and mono-crop coffee planting, which adversely affected the environment.

Bellanatonio and Yousefi (2016), examining the spread of soy cultivation in South America, expand upon the resulting switch in social reproduction:

For this investigation, we visited 28 sites across 3000 kilometers in Brazil and Bolivia, where soy production on an industrial scale is fueling massive deforestation... To overcome Burger King's lack of transparency, we used satellite mapping, supply chain analysis tools, interviews with soy growers and an extensive field investigation to uncover deforestation linked to agribusiness giants in the company's supply chain.

Across the South American frontier, we found the footprint of the major trading companies that sit astride global agriculture and supply Burger King and other food companies. Traders like the American companies Cargill, Bunge, and ADM buy grain, build silos and roads, provide farmers with fertilizer, and even finance land-clearing operations.

The resulting destruction, reversing recent declines in deforestation (Hecht 2014), can be reflected in global markets (and vice versa). Figure 1.2, adapted from Barona et al. (2010), shows the correlation coefficient between Amazon deforestation from 1995 to 2007 and the prices of soy and cattle. Correlation coefficients were centered on a moving average and a 9-year window, with price data leading deforestation by 1 year. Deforestation and soy prices appear increasingly integrated.

The environmental effects of such a switch in social reproduction can be seen from space. Figure 1.3, adapted from Tabuchi and Rigby (2017), shows satellite images of deforestation in a typical region of Brazil for 1984, 2000, and 2016. Brannstrom (2009, Lapola et al. 2014) situates similar maps for Western Bahia as the leading edge of Brazil's "neoliberal frontier":

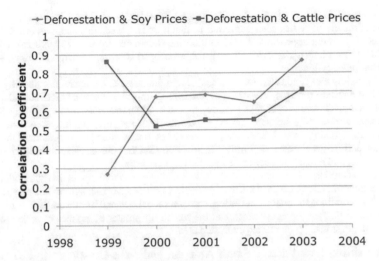

Fig. 1.2 Correlation coefficient over time between the prices of soy and cattle and Amazon deforestation from 1995 to 2007. Correlation coefficients were centered on a moving average and a 9-year window, price data leading deforestation by 1 year (adapted from Barona et al. 2010)

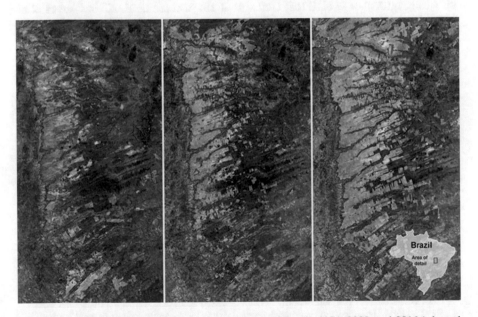

Fig. 1.3 Typical pattern of deforestation in one region of Brazil: 1984, 2000, and 2016 (adapted from Tabuchi and Rigby 2017)

Western Bahia is part of the ≈2 million km-sq. grassland - woodland Cerrado, of which approximately 55% has been converted to ranch or farmland. In 2006, western Bahia's cropland covered approximately 1.5 million ha, dominated by soy (850,000 ha), cotton (250,000 ha), and maize (166,000 ha), followed by 60,000 ha of irrigated crops under central-pivot systems...

By nearly every indicator, western Bahia is a quintessential neoliberal frontier. Soy area increased from nil in the late 1970s to 400,000 ha in 1988. By 1991, 182 central-pivot irrigation plots were in operation, and there would be more than 600 central-pivots by 2005. Farmers are strongly oriented toward export markets for soy, cotton, coffee, and fruit crops... Beginning around 2000, the government of Bahia extended modest subsidies for cotton and irrigated coffee and fruit - mainly infrastructure cost-sharing, value-added tax discounts, and rebates on finance charges for large projects.

Farms are large, usually exceeding 1000 ha; single landholdings in excess of 5000 ha are common... Likely causes for Cerrado clearing include favorable agronomic, policy, and market conditions for cotton cultivation, strong regional demand by soy crushers for wood fuel (from Cerrado or Eucalyptus), and the search for greater economies of scale among individual farmers by increasing cultivated area.

Such shifts, found across South America and Asia (Austin et al. 2017), have profound effects on vector epidemiology. Capital-led smoothing and "economies of scale" are having impacts on disease propagation across a range of pathogen taxa, including *Plasmodium*, *Leishmaniasis*, hantavirus, trypanosomatids, and even plant viruses (Gottdenker et al. 2012; Gottwalt 2013; Saccaro et al. 2016; Chaves et al. 2008; Roossnick and Garcia-Arenal 2015; Fornance et al. 2016). A large literature has identified the qualitative dynamics linking deforestation more specifically to vector-borne disease transmission dynamics across locale and pathogen (de Castro et al. 2006; Singer and de Castro 2001; Vasconcelos et al. 2006; Yasuoka and Levins 2007; Vittor et al. 2006, 2009; Fornace et al. 2016). Vittor et al. (2006) report:

[In the Peruvian Amazon] deforested sites had an *An. darlingi* biting rate that was more than 278 times higher than the rate determined for areas that were predominantly forested. Our results indicate that *An. darlingi* displays significantly increased human-biting activity in areas that have undergone deforestation and development associated with road development.

Olson et al. (2010) expand upon the observation using data from Brazil:

Our cross-sectional study shows malaria incidence across health districts in 2006 [for Mancio Lima County, Brazil] is positively associated with greater changes in percentage of cumulative deforestation within respective health districts... The landscape establishes local ecology and biodiversity, and our results confirm that cleared land is associated with higher malaria risk... Human malaria risk is specifically associated with deforestation 5–10 years previously...[in agreement] with other research that observed that shrub land cover, which develops 5 years after deforestation and becomes classified as secondary growth ≈ 15 years after deforestation, has significantly greater abundance of *An. darlingi* larvae than does forested land...[suggesting] that entomological risk is based on the fate of cleared land.

Populations of *Aedes aegypti* arise by a more urbanized niche construction, "produced," as medical entomologists describe it, in artificial containers connected to human management of water or, in the case of structural adjustment, declines in such public services (Barrera et al. 1995; 2011; Cox et al. 2007; Brown et al. 2014; Kraemer et al. 2015).

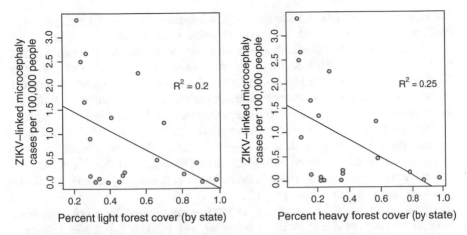

Fig. 1.4 Confirmed Zika-linked microcephaly cases in Brazilian states as a function of percent light and heavy forest cover. For a bivariate correlation of such a complex system, the relations are strongly negative: more forest cover, less pathology (from Ali et al. 2017)

A shift in mosquito community ecology on the heavily populated coast of Brazil was reported in 2000, with the arrival of *Aedes albopictus* in the native rain forests of Recife (de Albuquerque et al. 2000), the initial urban epicenter for Zika microcephaly, in what would be the heavily hit state of Pernambuco. *Ae. albopictus* joined already established major vector species such as *Ae. aegypti* and *Culex quinquefasciatus* and a diverse set of other and newly reported mosquito species here vectorially competent for the transmission of filariasis, dengue, Rocio, Mayaro virus, and yellow fever (Aragao et al. 2010; Carvalho et al. 2014).

The new epidemiologies appear driven by land use, even if for some diseases such shifts act only as proxies. Figure 1.4, from Ali et al. (2017), shows confirmed Zika-linked microcephaly cases in Brazilian states versus the percent of light and dense forest cover. Higher forest cover is strongly associated with lower case rates, a result comparable to that found in geospatial analyses of deforestation and Ebola outbreaks in West and Central Africa (Rulli et al. 2017). Even as the Zika outbreak in Latin America is primarily urban in scope, arriving from abroad by international travel and spreading city to city by the urban commuting field, the virus arrived in the middle of, and percolated through, a periurban gradient in vector epidemiology that in Zika's case appears tied to dengue and chikungunya dynamics (Faria et al. 2016a, b; Nah et al. 2016; Haque et al. 2016; Song et al. 2017).

With in vitro and indirect epidemiological data, Halstead et al. hypothesize Zika engages in reciprocal activation at the molecular level with dengue and perhaps yellow fever, which are clearly forest-dependent (Halstead 2003; Priyamvada et al. 2016; Kawiecki and Christofferson 2016; Cavalcanti et al. 2016; Halstead 2017; Mahalingam et al. 2017; Londono-Renteria et al. 2017). The convergent mutualism indicates that while Zika incidence is presently urban-driven, the virus is still associated with deforestation. Such ecological cascades are fundamentally relational, with disease dynamics in one locale dependent on those elsewhere. By a SIR model for nonhuman mammals, Althouse et al. (2016) meanwhile project a high probability Zika will revert to an endemic sylvatic ecotype in the Americas.

Other vector-borne infections appear similarly resurgent. An early census put nonhuman primate (NHP) deaths from an ongoing outbreak of yellow fever at 5000 in Southeastern Brazil alone, including the especially YF-sensitive northern brown howler monkey (*Alouatta guariba guariba*), the population-vulnerable northern masked titi monkey (*Callicebus personatus*), and the critically endangered northern muriqui (*Brachyteles hypoxanthus*) (Bicca-Marques et al. 2017). Forest fragmentation, isolating populations, appears to have reduced herd immunity even to sylvatic YF (Bicca-Marques and Freitas 2010; Oklander et al. 2017). NHP deaths across Latin America are estimated in the hundreds of thousands, threatening endangered species with extinction.

By a series of models, we next explore possible mechanisms by which capital-led land use and structural adjustment, intrinsically socialized into a single socioenvironmental object, drive vector-borne infection. Our line of formal argument, using stochastic generalizations of a classic disease model, aims to encapsulate the impacts of such disruptions in collective structures, technological shifts, expansions in highly capitalized farmland, road development, land-clearing operations, and rollbacks in municipal vector control on vector-borne infection. We show the results of this first line of modeling extend directly to more complex models.

References

Ali, S., Gugliemini, O., Harber, S., Harrison, A., Houle, L., et al., 2017, Environmental and social change drive the explosive emergence of Zika virus in the Americas, PLoS Neglected Tropical Diseases. doi: https://doi.org/10.1371/journal.pntd.0005135.

Althouse, B.M., Vasilakis, N., Sall, A.A., Diallo, M., Weaver, S.C., Hanley, K.A., 2016, Potential for Zika Virus to establish a sylvatic transmission cycle in the Americas, PLoS Negl Trop Dis, 10(12):e0005055.

Aragao, N.C., Muller, G.A., Balbino, V.Q., Costa Junior, C.R., Figueiredo Junior, C.S., Alencar, J., Marcondes, C.B., 2010, A list of mosquito species of the Brazilian State of Pernambuco, including the first report of Haemagogus janthinomys (Diptera: Culicidae), Yellow Fever vector and 14 other species (Diptera: Culicidae), Revista da Sociedade Brasileira de Medicina Tropical, 43(4):458–459.

Attaway, D.F., Waters, N.M., Geraghty, E.M., Jacobsen, K.H., 2017, Zika virus: Endemic and epidemic ranges of *Aedes* mosquito transmission, Journal of Infection and Public Health, 10(1):120–123.

Austin, K., Gonzalez-Roglich, M., Schaffer-Smith, D., Schwanes, A., Swenson, J., 2017, Trends in size of tropical deforestation events signal increasing dominance of industrial-scale drivers, Environmental Research Letters, 12:05–4009.

Ayres, C.F.J., 2016, Identification of Zika virus vectors and implications for control, Lancet Infect Dis, 16(3):278279.

Bailey, N.T.J., 1975, The Mathematical Theory of Infectious Diseases, Second Edition, Griffin, London.

Bailey, N.T.J., 1982, The Biomathematics of Malaria, Griffin, London.

Barona, E., Ramankutty, N., Hyman, G., Commes, O., 2010, The role of pasture and soybean in deforestation of the Brazilian Amazon, Environmental Research Letters, 5:024002.

Barrera, R., Amador, M., MacKay, A.J., 2011, Population dynamics of *Aedes aegypti* and dengue as influenced by weather and human behavior in San Juan, Puerto Rico, PLoS Negl Trop Dis, 5(12):e1378.

Barrera, R., Navarro, J.C., Mora, J.D., Dominguez, D., Gonzalez, J., 1995, Public service deficiencies and Aedes aegypti breeding sites in Venezuela, Bull Pan Am Health Organ., 29(3):193–205.

Bellanatonio, M., Yousefi, A., 2016. The ultimate mystery meat: Exposing the secrets behind Burger King and global meat production, Available online at www.mightyearth.org/mysterymeat/.

Bicca-Marques, J.C., Calegaro-Marques, C., Rylands, A.B., Strier, K., Mittermeirer, R., Almeida, M.A., et al., 2017, Yellow fever threatens Atlantic Forest primates, Sci. Adv. e-letter http://advances.sciencemag.org/content/3/1/e1600946/tab-e-letters.

Bicca-Marques, J.C., Freitas, D.S., 2010, The role of monkeys, mosquitoes, and humans in the occurrence of a yellow fever outbreak in a fragmented landscape in south Brazil: protecting howler monkeys is a matter of public health, Trop. Cons. Sci. 3:31–42.

Brannstrom, C., 2009, South America's neoliberal agricultural frontiers: Places of environmental sacrifice or conservation opportunity, AMBIO: A Journal of the Human Environment, 38(3):141–149.

Brown, J.E., Evans, B.R., Zheng, W., Obas, V., Barrera-Martinez, L., Egizi, A., Zhao, H., et al., 2014, Human impacts have shaped historical and recent evolution in *Aedes aegypti*, the dengue and yellow fever mosquito, Evolution, 68(2):514–525.

Carvalho, R.G., Loureno de Oliveira, R., Braga, I.A., 2014, Updating the geographical distribution and frequency of *Aedes albopictus* in Brazil with remarks regarding its range in the Americas, Memórias do Instituto Oswaldo Cruz, 109(6):787–796.

Cavalcanti, L.P., Tauil, P.L., Alencar, C.H., et al., 2016, Zika virus infection, associated microcephaly, and low yellow fever vaccination coverage in Brazil: is there any causal link?, J Infect Dev Cties, 10:563566.

Centeno, M.A., Cohen, J.N., 2012, The arc of neoliberalism, Annual Review of Sociology, 38:317340. doi: https://doi.org/10.1146/annurev-soc-081309-150235.

Chaves, L.F., 2017, Climate change and the biology of insect vectors of human populations. In: Johnson, S., Jones, H., editors, Invertebrates and Global Climate Change, Wiley, Chichester, UK, pp. 126–147.

Chaves, L.F., Cohen, J.M., Pascual, M., Wilson, M.L., 2008, Social exclusion modifies climate and deforestation impacts on a vector-borne disease, PLoS Neglected Tropical Diseases, 2(2):e176. Available online at https://doi.org/10.1371/journal.pntd.0000176.

Chaves, L.F. and Koenraadt, C.J.M., 2010, Climate change and highland malaria: Fresh air for a hot debate. The Quarterly Review of Biology, 85:27–55.

Chitunhu, S., Musenge, E. 2016, Spatial and socio-economic effects on malaria morbidity in children under 5 years in Malawi in 2012, Spatiotemporal Epidemiology 16:21–33.

Cover, T., Thomas, J., 2006, Elements of Information Theory, Second Edition, Wiley, New York.

Cox, J., Grillet, M.E., Ramos, O.M., Amador, M., Barrera, R., 2007, Habitat segregation of dengue vectors along an urban environmental gradient, Am J Trop Med Hyg., 76(5):820–826.

Dalal, N., Greenhalgh, D., Mao, X., 2007, A stochastic model of AIDS and condom use, Journal of Mathematical Analysis and Applications, 325:36–53.

de Albuquerque, C.M., Melo-Santos, M.A., Bezerra, M.A., Barbosa, R.M., Silva, D.F., da Silva, E., 2000, Primeiro registro de *Aedes albopictus* Area da Mata Atlantica, Recife, PE, Brasil, Revista de Saude Publica 34(3):314–315.

de Castro M., R. Monte-Mor, D. Sawyer, B. Singer, 2006, Malaria risk on the Amazon frontier, PNAS, 103:2452–2457.

Degeling, C., Johnson, J., Ian Kerridge, I., Andrew Wilson, A., Michael Ward, M., Cameron Stewart, C., Gwendolyn Gilbert, G., 2015, Implementing a One Health approach to emerging infectious disease: reflections on the socio-political, ethical and legal dimensions, BMC Public Health, 15:130.

Dick, G.W.A, Kitchen, S.F., Haddow, A.J. 1952, Zika Virus (I). Isolations and serological specificity, Transactions of the Royal Society for Tropical Medicine and Hygiene, 46(5):509–520.

Dzingirai, V., Bukachi, S., Leach, M., Mangwanya, L., Scoones, I., and Wilkinson, A., 2017, Structural drivers of vulnerability to zoonotic disease in Africa. Phil. Trans. R. Soc. B, 372(1725):20160169.

Evans, M.V., Dallas, T.A., Han, B.A., Murdock, C.C., Drake, J.M., 2017, Data-driven identification of potential Zika virus vectors, Elife, Feb 28;6. pii: e22053. doi: https://doi.org/10.7554/eLife.22053.

Faria, N.R., Azevedo Rdo, S., Kraemer, M.U., Souza, R., Cunha, M.S., Hill, S.C., Theze, J., 2016a, Zika virus in the Americas: Early epidemiological and genetic findings, Science, 352(6283):345–349.

Faria, N.R., Lourenco, J., Marques de Cerqueira, E., Maia de Lima, M., Pybus, O., Carlos Junior Alcantara, L., 2016b, Epidemiology of Chikungunya Virus in Bahia, Brazil, 2014-2015, PLoS Curr., 8, pii: ecurrents.outbreaks.c97507e3e48efb946401755d468c28b2

Faria, N.R., Quick, J., Claro, I.M., Theze, J., de Jesus, J.G., Giovanetti, M., Kraemer, M.U.G., et al., 2017, Establishment and cryptic transmission of Zika virus in Brazil and the Americas. Nature, 546:406–410.

Fernandes, R.S., Campos, S.S., Ferreira-de-Brito, A., de Miranda, R.M., da Silva, K.A.B., de Castro, M.G., et al., 2016, *Culex quinquefasciatus* from Rio de Janeiro is not competent to transmit the local Zika virus, PLoS Neglected Tropical Diseases, 10(9):e0004993.

Finley-Brook, M., 2007, Green neoliberal space: the Mesoamerican biological corridor, Journal of Latin American Geography, 6:101–124.

Fornace, K., Abidin, T., Alexander, N., Brock, P., Grigg, M., Murphy, A., William, T., et al., 2016, Association between landscape factors and spatial patterns of *Plasmodium knowlesi* infections in Sabah, Malaysia, Emerging Infectious Diseases, 22: doi: https://doi.org/10.3201/eid2202.150656.

Fornance, K., Abidin, T., Alexander, N., Brock, P. et al., 2016, Association between landscape factors and spatial patterns of *Plasmodium knowlesi* infections in Sabah, Malaysia, Emerging Infectious Diseases, 22, 201–208.

Ganti, T., 2014, Neoliberalism. Annual Review of Anthropology, 43:89104. doi: https://doi.org/10.1146/annurev-anthro-092412-155528.

Gottdenker, N., Chaves, L.F., Calzada, J.E., Saldana, A., Carroll, C.R., 2012, Host life history strategy, species diversity, and habitat influence *Trypanosoma cruzi* vector infection in changing landscapes, PLoS Negl Trop Dis, 6(11):e1884.

Gottwalt, A., 2013, Impacts of deforestation on vector-borne disease, Global Journal of Health Science, ghjournal.org/impacts-of-deforestation-on-vector-borne-disease-incidence-2/

Gray, A., Greenhalgh, D., Hu, L., Mao, X., Pan, J. 2011, A stochastic differential equation SIS epidemic model, SIAM Journal of Applied Mathematics, 71:876–902.

Halstead, S.B., 2003, Neutralization and antibody dependent enhancement of dengue viruses, Adv Virus Res., 60:421467.

Halstead, S.B., 2017, Biologic evidence required for Zika disease enhancement by dengue antibodies, Emerg Infect Dis., 23(4):569–573.

Haque, U., Ball, J.D., Zhang, W., Khan, M.M., Treviño, C.J.A., 2016, Clinical and spatial features of Zika virus in Mexico, Acta Trop., 162:5–10.

Harvey, D., 1982/2006, The Limits to Capital, Verso, New York.

Harvey, D., 2005, A Brief History of Neoliberalism, Oxford University Press, Oxford.

Hecht, S.B., 2014, Forests lost and found in tropical Latin America: the woodland 'green revolution', The Journal of Peasant Studies, 41(5):877–909.

Huddell, A., 2010, Effects of neoliberal reforms on small-scale agriculture in Brazil, Global Majority E-Journal, 1:74–84.

Hunter, F.F., 2017, Linking only *Aedes aegypti* with Zika Virus has world-wide public health implications, Front Microbiol., 8:1248.

Jones, B.A., Grace, D., Kock, R., Alonso, S., Rushton, J., Said, M.Y., et al., 2013, Zoonosis emergence linked to agricultural intensification and environmental change, PNAS, 110:8399 8404.

Jones, B.A., Betson, M., Pfeiffer, D.U., 2017, Eco-social processes influencing infectious disease emergence and spread, Parasitology, 144(1):26–36.

Kawiecki, A.B., Christofferson, R.C., 2016, Zika virus-induced antibody response enhances dengue virus serotype 2 replication in vitro, Journal of Infectious Diseases, 214:1357–1360.

Kindhauser, M.K., Allen, T., Frank, V., Santhana, R.S., Dye, C., 2016, Zika: the origin and spread of a mosquito-borne virus, Bull World Health Organ. 1;94(9):675–686C.

Kingsley, P., Taylor, E.M., 2017, One Health: competing perspectives in an emerging field, Parasitology, 144(1):7–14.

Kock, R.A., 2010, The newly proposed Laikipia disease control fence in Kenya, In K. Ferguson, J. Hanks (eds.), Fencing Impacts: A Review of the Environmental, Social and Economic Impacts of Game and Veterinary Fencing in Africa with Particular Reference to the Great Limpopo and Kavango-Zambezi Transfrontier Conservation Areas, 7175. Pretoria Mammal Research Institute.

Kraemer, M., Sinka, M., Duda, K., Myline, A., Shearer, F., Barker, C., et al., 2015, The global distribution of the arbovirus vectors *Aedes aegypti* and *Ae. Albopictus,* eLIFE, 4:e08347 (online open access).

Lapola, D.M., Martinelli, L.A., Peres, C.A., Ometto, J.P.H.B., Ferreira, M.E., et al., 2014, Pervasive transition of the Brazilian land-use system, Nature Climate Change, 4:27–35.

Le Flohic, G., Porphyre, V., Barbazan, P., Gonzalez, J.P., 2013, Review of climate, landscape, and viral genetics as drivers of the Japanese encephalitis virus ecology, PLoS Negl Trop Dis., 7(9):e2208.

Levins, R., Awerbuch, T., Brinkmann, U., Eckardt, I., Epstein, P., Makhoul, N., de Possas, C.A., Puccia, C., Spielman, A. and Wilson, M.E., 1994, The emergence of new diseases, American Scientist, 82:52–60.

Lindsay, S., Birley, M., 2004, Rural development and malaria control in Sub-Saharan Africa. Ecohealth, 1:129–137.

Londono-Renteria, B., Troupin, A., Cardenas, J.C., Hall, A., Perez, O.G., Cardenas, L., Hartstone-Rose, A., Halstead, S.B., Colpitts, T.M., 2017, A relevant in vitro human model for the study of Zika virus antibody-dependent enhancement, J Gen Virol. Jul 8. doi: https://doi.org/10.1099/jgv.0.000833.

Maas, B., Karp, D.S., Bumrungsri, S., Darras, K., Gonthier, D., Huang, J.C., Lindell, C.A., et al., 2016, Bird and bat predation services in tropical forests and agroforestry landscapes. Biol Rev Camb Philos Soc., 91(4):1081–1101.

Mahalingam, S., Teixeira, M.M., Halstead, S.B., 2017, Zika enhancement: a reality check, Lancet Infect Dis., 17(7):686–688.

Mandal, S., Sakar, R., Sinha, S., 2011, Mathematical models of malaria – a review, Malaria Journal, 10/1/202 (online open access).

Maye, D., Dibden, J., Higgens, V. , Potter, C, 2012, Governing biosecurity in a neoliberal world: Comparative perspectives from Australia and the United Kingdom, Environment and Planning A, 44:150168.

Maye, D., Enticott, G., Naylor, R., Ilbery, B., Kirwan, J., 2014, Animal disease and narratives of nature: Farmers reactions to the neoliberal governance of bovine Tuberculosis, Journal of Rural Studies, 36:401410.

Messina, J., Kraemer, M., Brady, O., Pigott, D., Shearer, F., Weiss, D., et al., 2016, Mapping global environmental suitability for Zika virus, eLIFE 5:e15272 (online).

Mirowski, P., 2009, Postface: defining neoliberalism, In P. Mirowski, D. Plehwe (eds), The Road From Mont Pélerin: The Making of the Neoliberal Thought Collective, Harvard University Press, Cambridge.

Miyagi, I. and Toma, T., 1980, Studies on the mosquitoes in Yaeyama Islands, Japan: 5. Notes on the mosquitoes collected in forest areas of Iriomotejima, Japanese Journal of Sanitary Zoology, 31:81–91.

Mogi, M. and Sota, T., 1996, Physical and biological attributes of water channels utilized by Culex pipiens pallens immatures in Saga City southwest Japan, Journal of the American Mosquito Control Association, 12:206–214.

Musso, D., 2015, Zika virus transmission from French Polynesia to Brazil, Emerging Infectious Disease, 21(10):1887.

Nah, K., Mizumoto, K., Miyamatsu, Y., Yasuda, Y., Kinoshita, R., Nishiura, H., 2016, Estimating risks of importation and local transmission of Zika virus infection, PeerJ., 4:e1904. doi: https://doi.org/10.7717/peerj.1904.

Oklander L.I., Miño, C.I., Fernández, G., Caputo, M., Corach, D., 2017, Genetic structure in the southernmost populations of black-and-gold howler monkeys (*Alouatta caraya*) and its conservation implications, PLos ONE, 12(10):e0185867.

Olson S., Gangnon, R., Silveira, G., Patz, J., 2010, Deforestation and malaria in Mancio Lima County, Brazil, Emerging Infection and Infectious Disease, 16:1108–1115.

Oviedo-Pastrana, M., Mendez, N., Mattar, S., Arrieta, G., Gomezcaceres, L., 2017, Epidemic outbreak of Chikungunya in two neighboring towns in the Colombian Caribbean: a survival analysis, Archives of Public Health, 75:1. doi: https://doi.org/10.1186/s13690-016-0169-1. eCollection 2017.

Priyamvada, L., Quicke, K.M., Hudson, W.H., et al., 2016, Human antibody responses after dengue virus infection are highly cross-reactive to Zika virus, Proc Natl Acad Sci USA, 113:78527857.

Protter, P., 1990, Stochastic Integration and Differential Equations, Springer, New York.

Roossinck, M., Garcia-Arenal, F., 2015, Ecosystem simplification, biodiversity loss and plant virus emergence, Current Opinion in Virology, 10:56–62.

Rosales-Castillo, J.A., Vazquez-Garciduenas, M.S., Alvarez-Hernandez, H., Chassin-Noria, O., Varela-Murillo, A.I., Zavala-Paramo, M.G., Cano-Camacho, H., Vazquez-Marrufo, G., 2011, Genetic diversity and population structure of *Escherichia coli* from neighboring small-scale dairy farms, J Microbiol., 49(5):693–702.

Rulli, M.R., Santini, M., Hayman, D.T.S, D'Odorico, P., 2017, The nexus between forest fragmentation in Africa and Ebola virus disease outbreaks, Scientific Reports, 7, Article number: 41613. doi: https://doi.org/10.1038/srep41613.

Saccaro, N., Mation, L., Sakowski, P., 2016, Impacts of deforestation on the incidence of diseases in the Brazilian Amazon, IPEA Discussion Paper 2145 (English ISSN 1415-4765) www.ipea.gov.br.

Samy, A.M., Thomas, S.M., Wahed, A.A., Cohoon, K.P., Peterson, A.T., 2016, Mapping the global geographic potential of Zika virus spread, Mem Inst Oswaldo Cruz, 111(9):559–560.

Schrecker, T., Bambra, C., 2015, How Politics Makes Us Sick: Neoliberal Epidemics, Palgrave MacMillan, New York.

Shen, S., Shi, J., Wang, J., Tang, S., Wang, H., Hu, Z., Deng, F. 2016. Phylogenetic analysis revealed the central roles of two African countries in the evolution and worldwide spread of Zika virus, Virol Sin., 31(2):118–130.

Singer, B., de Castro, M., 2001, Agricultural colonization and malaria on the Amazon frontier, Annals of the New York Academy of Sciences, 954:184–222.

Song, B.H., Yun, S.I., Woolley, M., Lee, Y.M. 2017, Zika virus: History, epidemiology, transmission, and clinical presentation, J Neuroimmunol. 308:50–64.

Tabuchi, H., Rigby, C., 2017, Amazon deforestation, once tamed comes roaring back, New York Times, Feb. 24, Times Business Day Online.

Tusting, L.S., Rek, J., Arinaitwe, E., Staedke, S.G., Kamya, M.R., Cano, J., Bottomley, C., et al., 2016, Why is malaria associated with poverty? Findings from a cohort study in rural Uganda, Infectious Disease and Poverty, 5(1):78.

Vasconcelos, C., Novo, E., Donalisio, M., 2006, Use of remote sensing to study the influence of environmental changes on malaria distribution in the Brazilian Amazon, Cad Saude Publica, 22:517–526.

Vittor, A., Gilman, R., Tielsch, J., Glass, G., Shields, T., Sanchez-Lozano, W., Pinedo-Cancino, V., Patz, J., 2006, The effects of deforestation on the human-biting rate of *Anopheles darlingi*, the primary vector of Falciparium Malaria in the Peruvian Amazon, American Journal of Tropical Medicine and Hugiene, 74:3–11.

Vittor, A., Gilman, R., Tielsch, J., Glass, G., Shields, T., Sanchez- Lozano, W., Pinedo, V., et al., 2009, Linking deforestation to Malaria in the Amazon: Characterization of the breeding habitat of the principal Malaria vector *Anopheles darlingi*, American Journal of Torpical Medicine and Hygiend, 81:5–12.

Wallace, R.G., Bergmann, L., Kock, R., Gilbert, M., Hogerwerf, L., Wallace, R., Holmberg, M., 2015, The dawn of Structural One Health: A new science tracking disease emergence along circuits of capital, Social Science and Medicine, 129:68–77.

Wallace, R.G., Kock, R.A., 2012, Whose food footprint? Capitalism, agriculture and the environment, Human Geography, 5(1):6383.

Wallace, R.G., Wallace, R. (eds.), 2016, Neoliberal Ebola: Modeling Disease Emergence from Finance to Forest and Farm, Springer, Switzerland.

Wang, W., Wenlong, L., Zizhen, L., Hui, Zhang, 2011, The effect of colored noise on spatiotemporal dynamics of biological invasion in a diffusive predator–prey system, Biosystems, 104(1):48–56.

Wilder-Smith, A., Gubler, D.J., Weaver, S.C., Monath, T.P., Heymann, D.L., Scott, T.W., 2017, Epidemic arboviral diseases: priorities for research and public health, Lancet Infect Dis. 17(3):e101–e106. doi: https://doi.org/10.1016/S1473-3099(16)30518-7.

Yang, H., Ferreira, M., 2000, Assessing the effects of global warming and local social and economic conditions on the malaria transmission, Revista de Saude Publica, 34:214–222.

Yang, Q., Mao, X., 2013, Extinction and recurrence of multi-group SEIR epidemic models with stochastic perturbations, Nonlinear Analysis: Real World Applications, 14:1434–1456.

Yasuoka, J., Levins, R., 2007, Impact of deforestation and agricultural development on anopheline ecology and malaria epidemiology, American Journal of Tropical Medicine and Hygiene, 76:450–460.

Zellweger, R.M., Cano, J., Mangeas, M., Taglioni, F., Mercier, A., Despinoy, M., Menks, C.E., et al., 2017, Socioeconomic and environmental determinants of dengue transmission in an urban setting: An ecological study in Nouma, New Caledonia. PLoS Neglected Tropical Diseases, 11(4):e0005471.

Chapter 2
Modeling Vector-Borne Diseases in a Commoditized Landscape

2.1 The Deterministic Approach

As Mandal et al. (2011) review, there is a rough hierarchy of models for vector-borne disease, focusing on malaria. These range from Ross (1911) through Macdonald (1957) to Anderson and May (1991), who present, respectively, two-, three-, and four-dimensional models. Macdonald and Anderson-May extend the Ross model to include latent periods in both human and vector. Further extensions explore the role of immune competence, superinfection, pathogen evolution, host and mosquito behavior, migration, population age structure, spatial dynamics, environmental factors, and so on, all largely variations on the Ross and Macdonald theme (Reiner et al. 2013). Yang (2000) studies a model containing ten differential equations.

Few such models consider socioeconomic factors, although Yang and Ferreira (2000) pursue a heroic attempt (see Mandal et al. 2011 for details) and Levins and Awerbuch-Friedlander tailor nonlinear difference models for public health policy and mosquito control (Predescu et al. 2007; Awerbuch-Friedlander and Levins 2009).

For our purposes, exploring causality in the socioeconomic field rather than solely in the objects of pathogen and vector, it is enough to examine and extend the simplest two-dimensional model, that of Ross. Following Bailey (1975), let X be the proportion of the human population that is infective and Y be the proportion of infective (female) mosquitoes. The deterministic epidemic equations are then

$$dX / dt = abmY(t)\left[1 - X(t)\right] - rX(t)$$
$$dY / dt = aX(t)\left[1 - Y(t)\right] - \mu Y(t)$$

(2.1)

where m is the number of female mosquitoes per human host, a is the number of bites per unit time on a host by a single mosquito, b is the proportion of infected bites on a host that produce an infection, r is the per capita rate of recovery in humans, and μ is the per capita mortality rate for mosquitoes.

The deterministic steady-state endemic levels, when $dX/dt = dY/dt = 0$, are

$$X_\infty = \frac{a^2 bm - \mu r}{a(abm + r)}$$

$$Y_\infty = \frac{a^2 bm - \mu r}{abm(a + \mu)}$$

(2.2)

If

$$a^2 bm \le \mu r$$

(2.3)

the endemic level is zero, and initial outbreaks will collapse.

Based on the qualitative observations of the previous sections, it is possible to make a simple deterministic model of the effects of smoothing on the infection steady state. Let ρ be an index of the degree of smoothing, in this case of deforestation or cuts in environmental sanitation, in a region where vector-borne infection had originally been driven to local near-extinction. For Eq. (2.1) we take $\mu = b = r = 1$ and $a = m = \rho + 1$. Then the relation for the proportion of the host population ultimately infected becomes

$$X_\infty(\rho) = \frac{(\rho+1)^3 - 1}{(\rho+1)\left[(\rho+1)^2 + 1\right]} \to 1$$

(2.4)

producing Fig. 2.1.

Our ultimate interest, however, is in the dynamics of transitions from low-level endemic to recurrent outbreak and particularly in the structure of imposed "noise" that might drive outbreaks to extinction or escape. That is, there is more here than the "endemicity" relation of Eqs. (2.2) and (2.3), so we need to explore the effects of noise by simulation.

2.2   Adding "Noise" to the Deterministic Model

We begin by setting $a = b = m = r = 1$ and $\mu = 0.9$ so that $X_\infty = 0.05, Y_\infty = 0.0526\ldots$

The basic equations follow

$$dX/dt = Y(t)\left[1 - X(t)\right] - X(t)$$

$$dY/dt = X(t)\left[1 - Y(t)\right] - 0.9Y(t)$$

(2.5)

Fig. 2.1 Steady-state proportion of human hosts infected vs. deforestation index for a region in which disease had been nearly eradicated. $\mu = r = b = 1$, $a = m = \rho + 1$. As ρ increases, $X\infty \to 1$

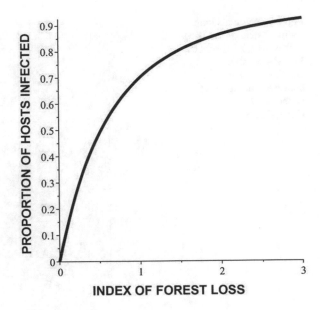

producing the "phase diagram" of Fig. 2.2, constructed from the DEplot function of the computer algebra program Maple 2016.

We next perturb the system with white noise and calculate the time dynamics using the ItoProcess function of Maple 2016. The simulation equations are

$$dX_t = \left(Y_t\left(1-X_t\right)-X_t\right)dt - 0.01Y_t dW_t^1$$
$$dY_t = \left(X_t\left(1-Y_t\right)-0.9Y_t\right)dt + 0.01X_t dW_t^2 \qquad (2.6)$$

where the dW_t^i are two white noise processes.

Figure 2.3 shows that for 30 simulations at low noise, the result is simply the expected S-shaped deterministic solution with some added diffusional "fuzz," and the system converges to near the deterministic endemic equilibrium.

Next, we add significant noise, with effects of differing sign:

$$dX_t = \left(Y_t\left(1-X_t\right)-X_t\right)dt - 0.4Y_t dW_t^1$$
$$dY_t = \left(X_t\left(1-Y_t-0.9Y_t\right)\right)dt + 0.4X_t dW_t^2 \qquad (2.7)$$

Figure 2.4 displays the result of 30 simulations. With sufficient added cross-noise of different signs, the system does not converge on the low deterministic endemic state but engages in repeated large excursions. Thus, while the "basic parameters" defining the low endemic level remain the same, added "noise" can still destabilize a public health system. The sequentially rising peaks are characteristic.

We need to emphasize that *all* models of two or more dimensions will inevitably suffer analogous explosive instabilities under appropriately structured and sufficiently large stochastic burden (Mao 2007; Appleby et al. 2008). Host-vector pathogen spread models are inherently at least two-dimensional in this sense.

Fig. 2.2 Phase diagram for the system of Eq. (2.5), with $X(0) = Y(0) = 0.001$. From these initial conditions, the system converges on the stable endemic state $(X = 0.05, Y = 0.053)$

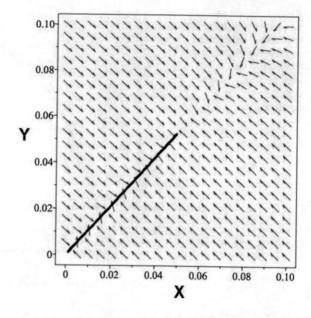

Fig. 2.3 Thirty simulations of Eq. (2.6) at cross-noise $= \pm 0.01$. The time development is just that of Eq. (2.5) plus some diffusion around the deterministic path. Red = X, blue = Y

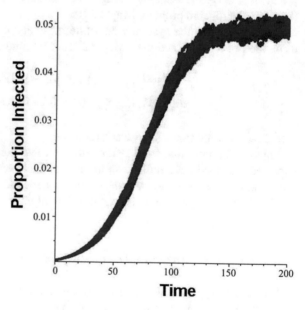

Fig. 2.4 The same as Fig. 2.3, but the cross-noise level is ±0.4, i.e., 40 times higher. The system diverges markedly from the low endemic level, generating repeated and increasing peaks of infection

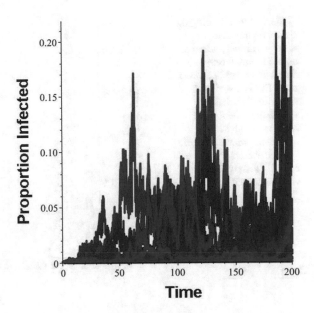

This is not the full story. The next simulation uses symmetric noise, having all positive signs, and is essentially the same as the Doléans-Dade exponential. The equations are

$$dX_t = \left(Y_t\left(1-X_t\right)-X_t\right)dt + 0.4X_t dW_t^1 + 0.4Y_t dW_t^2$$
$$dY_t = \left(X_t\left(1-Y_t\right)-0.9Y_t\right)dt + 0.4X_t dW_t^1 + 0.4Y_t dW^2$$

(2.8)

Figure 2.5, again for 30 simulations, shows the result. Individual outbreaks do not converge on the endemic level but fall to zero in the presence of sufficient symmetric stochasticity, as with the Ebola example and the Dole'ans-Dade exponential we explored in Chap. 1.

The inference is that for a vector-borne disease that is inherently at least two-dimensional as a consequence of the two basic populations of human and vector, the "wrong" noise – here of opposite signs – can blow up a low endemic level, while the "right" noise (large enough and all of positive sign) can collapse even low endemicity.

Real systems are likely to involve more than two interacting populations and indeed must address interacting geographic areas as well. Torres-Sorando and Rodriguez (1997) model two modes of malaria migration, migration with and without return, finding the equilibrium prevalence greater under the former. In a follow-up, Rodriguez and Torres-Sorando (2001) spatially partition subpopulations of hosts for vector-borne infection in one and two dimensions, with disease establishment easier under the latter. Gould and Wallace (1994) model a matrix of empirically collected human travel data between many multiple geographic subdivisions. Real systems can be of considerable dimensionality, a notion to which we will return.

Fig. 2.5 Reconfiguring the noise to symmetric sums – positively additive noise for both terms – drives the endemic level to zero. This is a standard result from stochastic stabilization theory and carries through to multidimensional dynamic systems even more complex than typical vector-borne disease

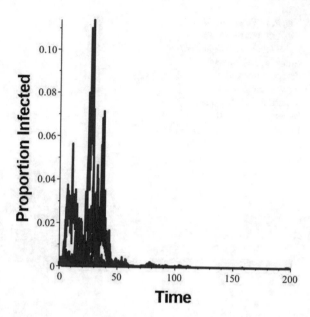

The mathematical mechanisms driving this contrary pattern for systems of two or more dimensions – one form of noise stabilizes, another form destabilizes – have only recently been addressed in the literature. We follow closely the explanation of Appleby et al. (2008).

2.3 Stochastic Stabilization and Destabilization

The mathematical gears turning behind the simulations of the previous section have been described for functions defined by both a global linear bound and, as a broader generalization, for *locally Lipschitz continuous*, that is, bounds set by a definite real number for which the absolute value of the slope of the line connecting every pair of points along the function does not exceed the real number (Mao 2007; Appleby et al. 2008).

More formally, a function $f(x)$ is said to be locally Lipschitz if, for f from $S \subset R^n \to R^m$, $m, n \geq 1$, there is a positive constant C such that

$$\|f(y) - f(x)\| \leq C \|y - x\| \tag{2.9}$$

for all $y \in S$ that are sufficiently near x. Appleby et al. (2008) then show that for any such f, a function g *can always be found* so that the perturbed stochastic differential equation

$$dX_t = f(X_t)dt + g(X_t)dW_t \tag{2.10}$$

either stabilizes an unstable equilibrium of f or, for dimensions ≥ 2, destabilizes a stable equilibrium. Here, dW_t is a multidimensional white noise. Scalar equations — one dimension — remain only stabilizable. Zika, malaria, and other vector-borne diseases are inherently at least two-dimensional, as they involve the interaction of host and vector populations.

Appleby et al. present what are in essence only existence equations – that under different conditions stabilization and destabilization are possible in a vector-borne pathogen growth. Moving from the mathematics, how does the destabilization Appleby et al. describe manifest in the biology of vector-borne systems?

We know how stochasticity can muffle pathogen population growth in one-dimensional systems: reducing the likelihood of lining up a series of hosts for extended transmission. The mechanisms by which agroeconomies impose pathogen destabilization in two-dimensional systems require further investigation.

In one possibility, spatial stochasticity may wobble the pathogen population into territories of previously untouched host populations, the continuous stochastic version of metapopulation rescue (Alonso et al. 2007; Adams and Kapan 2009; Simoes et al. 2008; Reluga 2016). The models we present to this point do not explicitly address space, but we hypothesize a demographic equivalent wherein nonoverlapping bursts of host and vector produce similar surges in pathogen growth. By a kind of passing stochastic resonance, a spike in vector should allow the pathogen to survive during a trough in host availability, and vice versa, with the worst of outbreaks timed to the convergence of host and vector population dynamics.

Other mechanisms appear possible.

Neoliberalism's lengthening commodity chains appear to increase the area over which pathogens and hosts interact, reducing the likelihood chance extirpation can drive an outbreak under replacement (lifting the disease system off its demographic floor). Phylogeography by Nelson et al. (2015) and Mena et al. (2016) shows wider reassortment in swine influenza (and faster evolution) associated with expanding international trade, including, for H1N1 (2009), the North American Free Trade Agreement (Wallace 2016a, b). In conjunction, such expansions increase the likelihood geographic searches for best fits of host and vector populations are successful, in this case flipping stochastically through combinations of environmental opportunity and vectoral capacity (Wallace and Wallace 2003; Wallace 2012).

Finally, there may be a socioeconomic Moran effect, wherein the dynamics of two separate populations become entrained by a shared exposure (Moran 1953; Hudson and Cattadori 1999; Chaves et al. 2012; Hening and Nguyen 2017). Empirically, the time correlation of the two populations converges on the correlation between the environmental variabilities where they live. The environmental noise both vector and host encounter may be (spatially) correlated (if also likely time-lagged), in this case perhaps tied to the kind of price-driven deforestation Barona et al. propose (Fig. 1.2) or any number of other empirically discoverable sources of anthropogenic effect (Liu et al. 2007; Hall and Turchin 2007; Rosenstock et al. 2011; Santos-Vega et al. 2016; Walter et al. 2017).

In the next section, we introduce a common framework under which several of these ostensibly divergent spatial mechanisms accelerate vector-borne outbreaks.

2.4   Stochastic Spatial Spread

The spatial spread of contagious processes – fads, rumors, and epidemics – has long been a central topic of quantitative geography (e.g., Hägerstrand 1967; Pyle 1969, 1979; Abler et al. 1971; Bailey 1975; Cliff et al. 1986; Gould 1993, 1999). Such phenomena, independent of exact mechanism, are typically driven by the embedding socioeconomic structures on and within which they take place. At different scales, these form the veritable riverbanks that channel the spatiotemporal dynamics of contagion and infection.

Typically geographers recognize three dominant processes acting at what are generally, but not always, progressively smaller scales: *hierarchical diffusion* nationally and internationally from larger to smaller conurbations along the travel patterns determined by roadways, railways, air, and river commerce. This is followed by *spatial diffusion* from central conurbations to surrounding settlements along daily travel routes, much like the spread of a wine stain on a tablecloth, and finally *network diffusion* along the social structures of personal day-to-day contact, for example, within a school, workplace, or family.

Case surveillance models and statistical phylogeographies have tracked the three processes in vector-borne diseases (e.g., Pham et al. 2016; Walter et al. 2016; Zhu et al. 2016; Haque et al. 2016; Zhang et al. 2017). As with other contagions, such outbreaks are historically bounded by prevalent modes of social reproduction and transportation. We see, for instance, recent shifts in the characteristic scale at which some vector-borne diseases are spreading (Noureddine et al. 2011; Gatherer and Kohl 2016). Clearly climate change and expanding travel networks are driving hierarchical diffusion at the global scale (Tatem et al. 2012; Huang et al. 2012; Rezza 2014), but shifts at regional scales also appear intimately tied to changing social geographies across periurban landscapes. Samson et al. (2015), for instance, document a change in mosquito distribution across five genera and ten species in Haiti. Prevalences in *Culex quinquefasciatus*, *Aedes albopictus*, and *Aedes aegypti* tracked rapid informal urbanization across agricultural, forest, and bare land post-earthquake, dynamics apparently associated with spikes in malaria.

Such epizootic shifts are by no means limited to neotropical forests or even non-industrial countries. The classic US example is that of tick-borne diseases, such as Lyme disease, other *Borrelia*, and human monocytic ehrlichiosis (Killilea et al. 2008; Raghavan et al. 2014; Salkeld et al. 2015). Deforestation, rural poverty, and the real estate bubbles of exurban development, the latter integrating disease ecologies across the sociospatial continuum, have changed the mix of interactions across primary and secondary hosts, including deer, mice, and opossum, not only expanding the interface between tick hosts and humans but in some cases also amplifying the force of infection (Ostfeld et al. 2006; Keesing et al. 2010).

The resulting surges in disease appear to arise from more than expansion in environments selecting for previously marginalized vectors. Ecotones themselves, the transition zones between ecologies, appear to select for a number of disease vector species, including mosquitoes, rodents, bats, pigs, ticks, and shellfish, leading to documented outbreaks in Sin nombre virus, yellow fever, Nipah, influenza, rabies, Lyme, cholera, leptospirosis, and malaria, among others (Despommier et al. 2006). Ecotones are dynamic and range across spatial scale from boundaries at the individual level up to the landscape level, including mosaics of patches varying in type, distance, and juxtaposition, with foundational impact upon biological productivity, genetic diversification, evolutionary trajectories, interspecific interactions, and dispersal of pathogens and vectors alike (e.g., Robertson et al. 2013; Raghavan et al. 2016).

As Despommier et al. (2006) describe, such cradles of evo-epidemiological innovation are entrained by human impact:

> It follows that ecotones include zones of interaction where large-scale land use change produces moving fronts where human settlements and accompanying cropland and pasture expand into relatively intact natural ecosystems. Such ecotones now dominate much of the geography of the world's tropical developing regions where land use change and forest conversion has been occurring at historically unprecedented rates in the past three decades... Human-created ecotones now extend across entire regions, superimposed on and expanding into natural ecotones, as well as extending deep into formerly intact blocks of continuous forest.

The scale effect of such a superimposition integrates ecosystems previously separated at the region level by both natural barriers and isolation by distance, with profound impact on disease dynamics. But to model such an effect, human interventions, giving even the most "natural" environments a social character, must be extended beyond notions of anthropogenic impact (Moore 2015; Davies 2016; Angus 2016; Foster and Burkett 2016; Kunkel 2017). As we touched on in the previous chapter, the effect, including upon disease, is instantiated by a particular moment in capitalist development (Wallace et al. 2015; Wallace and Wallace 2016).

Extractivist agro-industrial development, mining, livestock, land speculation, and infrastructure development, the factors driving major bouts of deforestation and disease emergence directly and indirectly, are embedded in state-supported global production networks and circuits of capital (DeFries et al. 2010; Lambin and Meyfroidt 2011; Bergmann and Holmberg 2016; Friis et al. 2016). The relationships between deforestation and land use are complex. In Brazil, land use changes associated with the agricultural sector, accounting for 20% of GDP, appear at one and the same time increasingly but not entirely decoupled from deforestation and increasing in intensification, consolidation, globalization, inequality, and speculation (Lapola et al. 2014; Rede Social de Justiça e Direitos Humanos et al. 2015; Oliveira 2016; Branford and Torres 2017) (Fig. 2.6a–d). Large-scale crops of pesticide-heavy, export-oriented soybean, sugarcane, and maize, and in pastures cattle, have driven expansions in commodity production, while smallholder staples such as rice, beans, and cassava have contracted (Pacheco and Poccard-Chapuis 2012; Meyfroidt et al. 2014; Fritz et al. 2015; Craviotti 2016; Oliveira 2016).

But the decline in the rate of deforestation, which in absolute terms continued to convert native vegetation into agropastoral land use, appears more recently to have been reversed or was never embarked upon elsewhere in South America (Austin et al. 2017). Barretto et al. (2013) meanwhile showed the relationship in Brazil to be

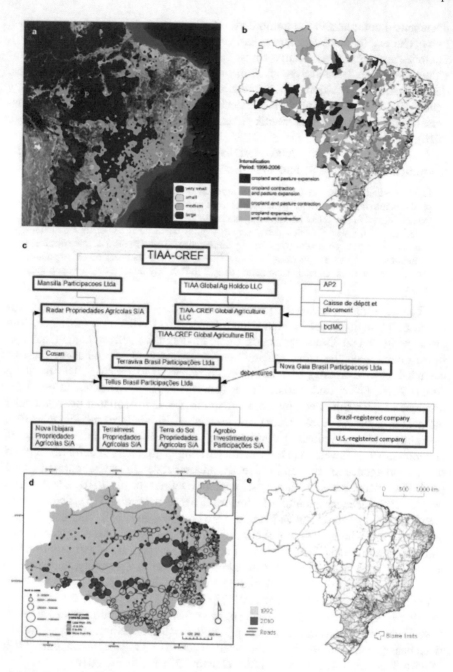

Fig. 2.6 Change in Brazilian land use. (**a**) Ranked field size based on 1 km global IIASA-IFPRI cropland percentage map for baseline year 2005 (Geo-Wiki Cropland, Fritz et al. 2015). (**b**) Combinations of expansion and contraction for cropland and pasture in minimum comparable areas where both crop production and pasture production intensified, 1996–2006 (Barretto et al. 2013). (**c**) Teachers Insurance and Annuity Association-College Retirement Equities Fund (TIAA-CREF)

geographically contingent. Increases in land use intensification in agriculturally consolidated areas coincided with contraction in both cropland and pasture or cropland expansion at the expense of pasture, while production on the forest frontier in central and northern Brazil coincided with expansion in cultivated land (Fig. 2.6b). The latter outcome instantiates the Jevons paradox, which in direct contradiction to the land sparing model offers a mechanism by which increasing efficiency of extraction, cheapening production, actually *increases* resource use and associated environmental destruction (Angelsen and Kaimowitz 2001; Ewers et al. 2009; Foster et al. 2010; Wallace and Kock 2012).

Concomitantly, "deforestation" is more than about trees. Commoditizing nature produces new ruralities, which even when in ostensible opposition to voracious deforestation reproduce colonialist regimes under new property models. NGO-led programs funded in part by publicity-sensitized agribusiness, what Hecht (2014) called green governance under a "junker" model, are defined by neoliberal logics around state-abetted "green" markets monetizing environmental services, offsets such as Reduced Emissions from Degradation and Deforestation (REDD+), boycotts for "environmental crimes," ecotourism, mass outmigration, and informalizing labor. Rural labor sensu lato – what turns the land into food – has been so devalued as to be maneuvered by the institutionalized competitive disadvantages of product and credit markets into compulsory transactions that upon near-usurious land sales turn farmers from owners to migrant wage labor or for the poorest toward the backbreaking, deproletarianized, and racialized "slave labor"of debt bondage (Taylor and García-Barrios 1999; Wright and Wolford 2003; McGarth 2013).

The resulting declines in forest destruction, never arrived upon in some areas and reversed in others, are encapsulated within a sphere of North-branded certification that helps inhibit traditional agroforest practices, expropriate smallholder pasture and cropland, promote farm consolidation and other economies of scale along Brannstrom's (2009) "neoliberal frontier," and rationalize passing the resulting overhead to depressed gate prices (which at the farm level selects for an increase in production further driving prices down). Among the many subsequent expansion pathways within this particular socioeconomic matrix, greenwashing the bigger brands, smallholders can be

---

Fig. 2.6 (continued) farmland investments in Brazil (Rede Social de Justiça e Direitos Humanos et al. 2015). The pension fund, now called just TIAA, is investing hundreds of millions in US$ into Brazilian fund Radar Propriedades Agrícolas S/A co-created with giant sugar producer Cosan to acquire land for sugarcane and other commodity crops. Cosan manages the fund, retaining first rights to acquire parcels before Radar, through TIAA's Brazilian subsidiary Mansilla Participacoes Ltda, and places them on the market. By 2012, Radar acquired 392 farms in Brazil of over 150,000 ha of an estimated value over US$1 billion. TIAA invests into Brazilian farmland by a second pathway: TIAA-CREF Global Agriculture LLC, a US$2 billion global farmland fund aimed at Australia, Brazil, and the USA. To circumvent Brazilian law against foreign acquisitions, TCGA invests indirectly through Tellus Brasil Participações Ltda., also managed by Cosan. (**d**) Dynamic agriculture frontier in Brazilian Legal Amazon: cattle population by municipality and along road infrastructure (Pacheco and Poccard-Chapuis 2012). (**e**) Urban areas as detected from nightlight glow, 1992 and 2010. Note the growing periurban infrastructure through ostensibly rural areas (Lapola et al. 2014)

displaced to deforestation's bleeding edge nearby or, if such land is locally unavailable, to distal edges in another state (Schmink 1994; Rosa et al. 2012; Chappell et al. 2013; Meyfroidt et al. 2014). Across these multiple effects, the green capitalism Northern consumers embrace replaces rural epistemes around which forest ecologies were previously organized (and were able to reproduce themselves in working landscapes to the mutual benefit of indigenous and nonhuman populations alike).

Declines in deforestation, then, are not synonymous with forest conservation. In this case, they appear entwined with an imperial projection of unequal ecological exchange, a recapitulation of the counterrevolutionary objectives of the Green Revolution, a deeper history of Malthusian rationalization, and a primitive accumulation by another name – "save the Earth" (Harvey 1982/2006; Freebairn 1995; Jorgenson 2006; Foster et al. 2010; Patel 2013; Chappell et al. 2013).

Hecht (2014) spatialized these transitions:

> Globalization and migration, whether regional or international, move peasant analysis away from the livelihood dynamics of a single locality...into complex scales and nodal flows rather than just an analysis of the dynamics of place... We don't even really have a name for what these sorts of rural dwellers are since the categories of urban-rural, agricultural-forest, local-regional and national-international are so intertwined.

Without discounting Oliveira's (2016) notion of the deeply embedded ties between the neoliberal state and Latin-American production and a Brazil-led, south-south sub-imperialism at odds with USA and EU hegemony, Turzi (2011) regionalized the associated commodities:

> National borders are losing ground to a corporate-driven model of territorial organization. The new model is dictating production conditions and infrastructural developments; rearranging the geoeconomic space throughout Argentina, Bolivia, Brazil, Uruguay, and Paraguay into a single, unified "Soybean Republic".

We have here no deterrorialization but, as Haesbaert (2011, Craviotti 2016) conceptualizes it, a reconfiguration into a multiscalar and spatially discontinuous network of fluctuating territorial embeddedness. The new multiterritoriality is reflected, as Jepson et al. (2010), Meyfroidt et al. (2014), and here Oliveira (2016) describe, in its management, capitalization, subcontracting, supply chain substitutions, leasing, and transnational land pooling:

> It becomes increasingly clear that Brazilian agribusiness leaders – and those in the soybean sector prominent among them – are new protagonists of global agroindustrial production networks and multilateral governance institutions. This follows upon a transformation of the very character of soybean farmers in Brazil (and Argentina). Unlike the entrepreneurial soybean family farmers from the Midwest of the U.S., the largest and most politically powerful Brazilian soybean farmers have expanded to the scale and organizational structure of veritable agribusiness enterprises: 'The classic image of poor farmers and rich ranchers is replaced by one of rural managers, most of them with university-level education, living in cities and specialized in business management. The MBAs are replacing farmers'...

As Craviotti (2016) summarizes it, such networks are flexibly embedded into non-contiguous biological and political territories, each node only opportunistically attentive to local needs and expectations, although at times they are forced to be, relying on area infrastructure or a small pool of brand-loyal contract smallholders for local expertise and social brokering. Contracting such co-operators place to place produces a "fractal" geography of networks of networks. The territories in turn are embedded into the networks.

Oliveira (2016) converges on the bet-hedging that Burch (2005) observes in horizontal multinational production, wherein glitches at one site are covered by fixes at another, but adds the financial speculation backing these food commodities. The housing bubble driving the Great Recession in the USA, for instance,

triggered in turn a sudden rush for farmland and agroindustrial investments that seeks to diversify production factors of agroindustrial commodities, thereby transforming both financial and ecological volatility from structural vulnerabilities to opportunities for windfall profits... In other words, expanding and broadening one's portfolio with transnational operations enables an agribusiness company (and financial institutions lending to or owning stocks in agribusiness companies) to make extra profits from its operations in Brazil, for example, when there are major droughts or financial crises in the U.S., and vice versa.

The Recession surge was no one-shot deal. Such speculation is codified in the regional and international credit and future markets backing agricultural producers in an increasingly volatile and lucrative sector. Such higher-order bets, Johnson (2013; Wallace 2016a, b) observed, have long bent agricultural commodities beyond their material qualifications as food or fuel sources delivered to global customers and toward their marketability, money valuation, and fungibility as defined by the needs of capital positioned elsewhere in space and portfolio. Distance, as Johnson puts it, is measured "not in miles, but in dollars." Perverse outcomes can prevail with virtual crops – annual debt payments, some packaged into derivatives – at times preempting a functional agricultural market, even well in advance of a season's planting.

McGarth (2013) meanwhile contemporized Johnson's industrial ecology of US slavery, matching the state of labor rights in Brazil to the change in production's spatial scale:

Those liberated from slave labour in sugar cane are generally agricultural workers, most commonly employed as seasonal workers in manual cane cutting. Most are internal migrants; while workers experience violations of labour and employment law, these are typically less severe among workers who are able to return home at the end of the day (or at least the end of the week). The origin of these migrant workers has changed over the years as the labour frontier...has shifted... The 23 slave labour cases occurred in the coastal Northeast (where sugar has been grown since the colonial era); in areas where there were few producers in the region (e.g., North/Northeast but not part of the coast regions); and in areas of expansion (e.g., Centre-West).

Despite a decade-long secular shift in population from commoditized rural areas to urban slums that continues today, the rural-urban dichotomy driving much of the discussion around vector-borne diseases misses this rural-destined labor and the rapid growth of rural towns into periurban *desakotas* (city villages) or *Zwishenstadt* (in-between cities), oft-acting as both local markets and regional hubs for global ag commodities passing through (Davis 2006; Hecht 2014) (Fig. 2.6e). Other countrysides have turned "post-agricultural" (Lugo 2009). Metropolitan regions meanwhile produce (some of) their own food, act as sources for rural land speculation, and act as sinks for the semi-proletarianized cycle migration that helps import rural consumption patterns (Padoch et al. 2008; Chappell 2018). The resulting informal influx overloads urban environmental sanitation, selecting for vector-borne outbreaks at this end of the periurban gradient (e.g., Caprara et al. 2009; Mota et al. 2016).

As Lerner and Eakin (2011) summarize:

Segmenting the landscape into urban and rural upholds a dichotomy that is increasingly obsolete. In many parts of the developing world, peri-urban landscapes reflect an organic spatial heterogeneity and multifunctionality that could be an untapped resource. In these spaces, there are unexplored opportunities for enhancing regional food security and, through the provision of a diversity of ecosystem services, environmental sustainability...

In visually 'rural' landscapes, the footprint of industry nearby is reflected in polluted groundwater and the profile of household incomes. The fusion of livelihoods is seen along apparently urban streets, where livestock and gardens occupy back patios, and the younger generations commute to the locations of their professional careers. In this hybrid landscape, land use and livelihood change are in constant tension.

Such geographies affect disease. Cuong et al. (2013), for instance, reported dengue incidence, typically thought an urban disease, to be synchronized with a characteristic area entraining Ho-Chi Minh City's periurban and rural environs out to 50–100 km. Guagliardo et al. (2014, 2015) found urban vector *Aedes aegypti* in the surrounding rural areas out to 19 km from Iquitos, the largest city in the Peruvian Amazon. Fonzi et al. (2015) found low genetic structure in *Ae. aegypti* across seven major islands of central-western Philippines, particularly across busy ports. Cargo shipments appeared a primary mode of spread in both Peru and the Philippines.

Sylvatic dynamics are no longer constrained to the hinterlands alone. Their associated epidemiologies are similarly relational. Almost all the mechanisms proposed at the end of the previous section explaining how stochasticities can drive two-dimensional epidemiologies of host and vector – metapopulation rescue, stochastic resonance, geographic search, and the Moran effect – centered upon the shifting scales at which outbreaks now spread across restructured landscapes, commuting fields, and commodity webs.

Structural One Health need now include what Moench and Gyawali (2008) call a "desakota science": Are some commodities and their market, investment, tax, subsidy, banking, infrastructure, transport, and labor contexts (Angelsen and Kaimowitz 2001; Pacheco and Poccard-Chapuis 2012; Meyfroidt et al. 2014) more associated with land uses that favor specific vector-borne outbreaks over others? Are some metapopulation structures produced across such commodity networks and periurban ecotones more supportive of endemicity or the evolution of pathogen virulence than others? Carvalho et al. (2009), for instance, reported landscapes dominated by crops to be more fragmented than when dominated by pastures. What is the epidemiology that arises out of production organized around, as one company conceptualized it, "yields with no borders," albeit structured by a new set of territorialities and the dynamic relative positions of the different social groups and vectors in them (Harvey 1982/2006; Craviotti 2016)?

How might we start to assimilate such a complex, fractal geography?

Much previous work on the geographic diffusion of HIV/AIDS in the USA was, at base, deterministic although framed by probability-of-contact matrices across conurbations at different scales and levels of organization (e.g., Wallace et al. 1997, 1999; Gould and Wallace 1994). Here, we will extend that work to study the effects of "noise" and policy-driven smoothing, consistent with the analyses of the previous sections. Emerging infections – including the vector-borne – that are not "slow plagues" with long, asymptomatic infection periods as in HIV/AIDS will be expressed rapidly across much smaller geographic and social venues, providing opportunities for stochastic effects that, in the absence of "smoothing" policies, can drive emerging spatiotemporal dynamics to extinction (Wallace 2017a, b).

Following Gould and Wallace (1994), the spread of a "signal" on a particular network of interacting geographic sites – between and within – is described at non-equilibrium steady state in terms of an equilibrium distribution ε_i "per unit area" A_i of a Markov process, where the A_i scale with the different "size" of each node, taken as distinguishable by the scale variable A_i as well as by its "position" i or the associated probability of contact matrix (POCM). The POCM is then normalized to a stochastic matrix $\mathbf{Q}$ having unit row sums, and the vector ε calculated as $\varepsilon = \varepsilon\mathbf{Q}$.

There is a vector set of dimensionless network flows $X_{t\,i}$, $i = 1, ..., n$ at time t. These are each determined by some relation:

$$X_t^i = g\left(t, \varepsilon_i / A_i\right) \tag{2.11}$$

Here, i is the index of the node of interest, $X_{t\,i}$ the corresponding dimensionless scaled i-th signal, t the time, and g an appropriate function. Again, ε_i is defined by the relation $\varepsilon = \varepsilon\mathbf{Q}$ for a stochastic matrix $\mathbf{Q}$, calculated as the network probability-of-contact matrix between regions, normalized to unit row sums. Using $\mathbf{Q}$, we have broken out the underlying network topology, a fixed between-and-within travel configuration weighted by usage that is assumed to change relatively slowly on the time scale of observation compared to the time needed to approach the nonequilibrium steady-state distribution.

Since the X are expressed in dimensionless form, g, t, and A_i must be rewritten as dimensionless as well giving, for the monotonic increasing function F

$$X_\tau^i = G\left[\tau, \frac{\varepsilon_i}{A_i} \times A_\tau\right] \tag{2.12}$$

where A_τ is the value of a characteristic area variate that represents the spread of the perturbation signal at (dimensionless) characteristic time $\tau = t/T_0$.

G may be quite complicated, including dimensionless "structural" variates for each individual geographic node i. The idea is that the characteristic "area" A_τ grows according to a stochastic process, even though G may be a deterministic mix master driven by systematic local probability-of-contact or flow patterns.

We offer a simple example.

A characteristic area of an outbreak cannot grow indefinitely, and we invoke a "carrying capacity" for the geographic network under study, say $K > 0$. An appropriate stochastic differential equation is then

$$dA_\tau = \left[\mu\rho A_\tau\left(1 - A_\tau / K\right)\right]d\tau + \sigma A_\tau dW_\tau \tag{2.13}$$

where we take ρ as representing a policy-driven "smoothing" index across an initially highly irregular mosaic enterprise, subdivided by dynamic land use mode, punctuated time frames, and so on.

Using the Itô chain rule on $\log(A)$, as a consequence of the added Itô correction factor and the Jensen inequality for a concave function,

$$E(A) \to 0, \mu\rho < \sigma^2/2$$

$$E(A) \geq K\left(1 - \frac{\sigma^2}{2\mu\rho}\right), \mu\rho \geq \sigma^2/2 \tag{2.14}$$

Figure 2.7 shows the form of this relation.

While zero is an attainable stochastic limit of the characteristic area below the critical smoothing value, above that, the infection becomes endemic and, as smoothing increases, may attain its greatest possible value as a pandemic.

The central inference, then, is that neoliberal or colonial smoothing of "outback" land use practices will cause sporadic disease outbreaks that would die out rapidly and be limited geographically to become either endemic or of significant spatial extent. Such, in turn, are entrained into larger travel patterns and deposited in central places, where they incubate and then spread explosively down and across social and economic hierarchies.

We can apply such an inference to more specific hypotheses.

We might propose, for instance, an epidemiological equivalent to recent efforts at debunking Forest Transition Theory (FTT) and its associated environmental Kuznets curves (EKC). FTT and EKC assert a country's environmental footprint rises and then declines with its economic development. Wealth from agriculture drives industrialization, attracting people to the city as to let rural areas regenerate. Setting aside the dearth of data in support of EKC (Mills and Waite 2009; Choumert et al. 2013; Bergmann 2017) and FTT's dubious theoretical underpinnings (Perfecto and Vandermeer 2010), Mansfield et al. (2010) show declines in deforestation in actuality are dependent on the global North's capacity to import forest and agricultural products – and export the attendant environmental damage – when its economies are booming.

We can similarly hypothesize a reverse Forest Transition Theory for disease: vector-borne pathogens associated with globalized agriculture commodities emerge and spread at scale on global commodity webs when demand from the global north increases. Such a hypothesis, open to empirical investigation, is likely to be at best a first-order approximation, as diseases emerge for a variety of context-specific reasons. But it is the relational nature of such a model of disease ecology, extending to even the other side of the world, that should spur new lines of research (Wallace et al. 2015; Friis et al. 2016). We will return to such a research program in the final chapter.

But by any of these mechanisms driving vector-borne outbreaks, if disease outcomes are context-driven, emerging more than merely out of the specifics of exposure and infection, then successful interventions must extend well beyond individualist, and even small-area, prophylaxes, however necessary these remain.

Fig. 2.7 Lower limit of the expectation for the characteristic area of a spreading infection as a function of a policy-driven smoothing measure, i.e., "economies of scale" that increase the sizes of units of production and the scales of commodity and labor webs across the periurban continuum

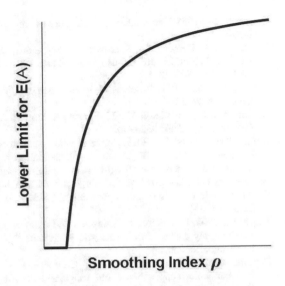

The latter only recapitulate the ideology behind the market atomization driving the outbreaks to begin with (Wallace et al. 2015). But what, as Dzingirai et al. (2017) ask, drives the drivers? In the next chapter, we explore an alternate approach to both characterizing and intervening into disease outbreaks.

References

Abler, R., Adams, J., Gould, P., 1971, Spatial Organization: The Geographer's View of the World, Prentice Hall, New York.

Adams, B, Kapan, D.D., 2009, Man bites mosquito: understanding the contribution of human movement to vector-borne disease dynamics, PLoS One, 4(8):e6763. doi: https://doi.org/10.1371/journal.pone.0006763.

Alonso, D., McKane, A.J., Pascual, M., 2007, Stochastic amplification in epidemics, J R Soc Interface, 4(14):575–582.

Anderson, R., May, R., 1991, Infectious Diseases of Humans: Dynamics and control, Oxford University Press, London.

Angelsen, A., Kaimowitz, D., 2001, Agricultural Technologies and Tropical Deforestation, CAB International, Wallingford, UK.

Angus, I., 2016, Facing the Anthropocene: Fossil Capitalism and the Crisis of the Earth System, Monthly Review Press, New York.

Appleby, J., Mao, X., Rodkina, A., 2008, Stabilization and destabilization of nonlinear differential equations by noise, IEEE Transactions on Automatic Control, 53:126–132.

Appleby, J., Mao, X., Rodkina, A., 2008, Stabilization and destabilization of nonlinear differential equations by noise, IEEE Transactions on Automatic Control, 53:683–691.

Austin, K., Gonzalez-Roglich, M., Schaffer-Smith, D., Schwanes, A., Swenson, J., 2017, Trends in size of tropical deforestation events signal increasing dominance of industrial-scale drivers, Environmental Research Letters, 12:05–4009.

Awerbuch-Friedlander, T., Levins, R. 2009, Mathematical models of public health, In J.A. Filar, J.B. Krawczyk (eds), Encyclopedia of Life Support Systems: Mathematical Models 3 /EOLSS Publishers/UNESCO, Singapore.

Bailey, N.T.J., 1975, The Mathematical Theory of Infectious Diseases, Second Edition, Griffin, London.

Barretto, A.G., Berndes, G., Sparovek, G., Wirsenius, S, 2013, Agricultural intensification in Brazil and its effects on land-use patterns: an analysis of the 1975- 2006 period, Glob Chang Biol., 19(6):1804–1815.

Bergmann, L.R., 2017, Towards economic geographies beyond the Nature-Society divide, Geoforum, 85:324–335.

Bergmann, L.R., Holmberg, M., 2016, Land in motion, Annals of the American Association of Geographers, 106(4):932–956.

Branford, S., Torres, M., 2017, Amazon land speculators poised to gain control of vast public lands, Mongabay, 27 March. Available online at https://news.mongabay.com/2017/03/amazon-land-speculators-poised-to-gain-control-of-vast-public-lands/.

Brannstrom, C., 2009, South America's neoliberal agricultural frontiers: Places of environmental sacrifice or conservation opportunity, AMBIO: A Journal of the Human Environment, 38(3):141–149.

Burch, D., 2005, Production, consumption and trade in poultry: Corporate linkages and North-South supply chains., In N. Fold and W. Pritchard (eds), Cross- Continental Food Chains, Routledge, London, pp 16678.

Caprara, A., Lima, J.W., Marinho, A.C., Calvasina, P.G., Landim, L.P., Sommerfeld, J., 2009, Irregular water supply, household usage and dengue: a bio-social study in the Brazilian Northeast, Cad Saude Publica., 25 Suppl 1:S125–S136.

Carvalho, F.M.V., De Marco Ju´nior, P., Ferreira, L.G., 2009, The Cerrado into pieces: Habitat fragmentation as a function of landscape use in the savannas of central Brazil, Biological Conservation, 142(7):1392–1403.

Chappell, M.J., 2018, Beginning to End Hunger: Food and the Environment in Belo Horizonte, Brazil, and Beyond, University of California Press, Berkeley.

Chappell, M.J., Wittman, H., Bacon, C.M., Ferguson, B.G., Barrios, L.G., Barrios, R.G., Jaffee, D., Lima, J., Méndez, V.E., Morales, H., Soto-Pinto, L., Vandermeer, J., Perfecto, I., 2013, Food sovereignty: an alternative paradigm for poverty reduction and biodiversity conservation in Latin America, F1000Res, 2:235.

Chaves, L.F., Satake, A., Hashizume, M., Minakawa, N., 2012, Indian Ocean dipole and rainfall have a Moran effect in East Africa malaria transmission, Journal of Infectious Diseases, 205:1885–1891.

Choumert, J., Moteland, P.C., Dakpo, H.K., 2013, Is the environmental Kuznets curve for deforestation a threatened theory? A meta-analysis of the literature, Ecological Economics, 90:1928.

Cliff, A., P. Haggett, J. Ord, 1986, Spatial Aspects of Influenza Epidemics, Pion, London.

Craviotti, C., 2016, Which territorial embeddedness? Territorial relationships of recently internationalized firms of the soybean chain, The Journal of Peasant Studies, 43(2):331–347.

Cuong, H.Q., Vu, N.T., Cazelles, B., Boni, M.F., Thai, K.T.D., Rabaa, M.A., Quang, L.C., Simmons, C.P., Huu, T.N., Anders, K.L., 2013, Spatiotemporal dynamics of dengue epidemics, Southern Vietnam, Emerg Infect Dis., 19(6):945953.

Davies, J., 2016, The Birth of the Anthropocene, University of California Press, Berkeley.

Davis, M., 2006, Planet of Slums, Verso, New York.

DeFries, R.S., Rudel, T.K., Uriarte, M., Hansen, M., 2010, Deforestation driven by urban population growth and agricultural trade in the twenty-first century, Nat. Geosci., 3:17881.

Despommier, D., Ellis, B.R., Wilcox, B.A., 2006, The role of ecotones in emerging infectious diseases, Ecohealth, 3(4):281–289.

Dzingirai, V., Bukachi, S., Leach, M., Mangwanya, L., Scoones, I., and Wilkinson, A., 2017, Structural drivers of vulnerability to zoonotic disease in Africa. Phil. Trans. R. Soc. B, 372(1725):20160169.

Ewers, R.M., Scharlemann, J.P.W., Balmford, A., et al., 2009, Do increases in agricultural yield spare land for nature? Glob Change Biol., 15(7):17161726.

Fonzi, E., Higa, Y., Bertuso, A.G., Futami, K., Minakawa, N., 2015, Human-mediated marine dispersal influences of the population structure of *Aedes aegypti* in the Philippine archipelago, PLoS Neglected Tropical Diseases, 9(6):e0003829.

Foster, J.B., Burkett, P., 2016, Marx and the Earth: An Anti-Critique, Brill, The Netherlands.

Foster, J.B., Clark, B., York, R., 2010, The Ecological Rift: Capitalism's War on the Earth, Monthly Review Press, New York.

Freebairn, D.K., 1995, Did the Green Revolution concentrate incomes? A quantitative study of research reports. World Dev., 23(2):265279.

Friis, C., Nielsena, J.Ø., Oteroa, I., Haberla, H., Niewöhnera, J., Hostert, P., 2016, From teleconnection to telecoupling: taking stock of an emerging framework in land system science, Journal of Land Use Science, 11(2):131153.

Fritz, S., See, L., McCallum, I., Bun, A., Moltchanova, E., Dürauer, M., Perger, C., Havlik, P., et al., 2015, Mapping global cropland field size, Global Change Biology, 21(5):1980–1992.

Gatherer, D., Kohl, A., 2016, Zika virus: a previously slow pandemic spreads rapidly through the Americas, J Gen Virol. 97(2):269–273.

Gould, P., 1993, The Slow Plague, Blackwell, Oxford, UK.

Gould, P., 1999, Becoming a Geographer, Syracuse University Press, Syracuse NY.

Gould, P., R. Wallace, 1994, Spatial structures and scientific paradox in the AIDS pandemic, Geografiska Annaler, 76B:105–116.

Guagliardo, S.A., Barboza, J.L., Morrison, A.C., Astete, H., Vazquez-Prokopec, G., Kitron, U., 2014, Patterns of geographic expansion of *Ades agypti* in the Peruvian Amazon, PLoS Neglected Tropical Diseases, 8(8):e3033.

Guagliardo, S.A., Morrison, A.C., Barboza, J.L., Requena, E., Astete, H., Vazquez- Prokopec, G., Kitron, U., 2015, River boats contribute to the regional spread of the dengue vector *Aedes aegypti* in the Peruvian Amazon, PLoS Neglected Tropical Diseases, 9(4):e0003648.

Haesbaert, R., 2011, El mito de la desterritorialización. Del fin de los territorios a la multiterritorialidad. México: Siglo XXI.

Hägerstrand, T., 1967, Innovation Diffusion as a Spatial Process, University of Chicago Press, Chicago.

Hall, T.D., Turchin, P., 2007, Lessons from population ecology for World-Systems analyses of long-distance synchrony, In A. Hornberg, C.L. Crumley (eds) The World System and the Earth System: Global Socioenvironmental Change and Sustainability Since the Neolithic, Left Coast Press, Walnut Creek, CA, pp 74–90.

Haque, U., Ball, J.D., Zhang, W., Khan, M.M., Treviño, C.J.A., 2016, Clinical and spatial features of Zika virus in Mexico, Acta Trop., 162:5–10.

Harvey, D., 1982/2006, The Limits to Capital, Verso, New York.

Hecht, S.B., 2014, Forests lost and found in tropical Latin America: the woodland 'green revolution', The Journal of Peasant Studies, 41(5):877–909.

Hening A, Nguyen, D.H., 2017, Stochastic Lotka-Volterra food chains, arXiv:1703.04809.

Huang, Z., Das, A., Qiu, Y., Tatem, A.J., 2012, Web-based GIS: the vector-borne disease airline importation risk (VBD-AIR) tool, Int J Health Geogr., 11:33.

Hudson, P.J., Cattadori, I.M., 1999, The Moran effect: a cause of population synchrony, Trends in Ecology & Evolution, 14(1):1–2.

Jepson, W., Brannstrom, C., Filippi, A., 2010, Access regimes and regional land change in the Brazilian Cerrado, 1972 - 2002, Annals of the Association of American Geographers, 100(1):87–111.

Johnson, W., 2013, River of Dark Dreams: Slavery and Empire in the Cotton Kingdom, Harvard University Press, Cambridge, MA.

Jorgenson, A.K., 2006, Unequal ecological exchange and environmental degradation: a theoretical proposition and cross-national study of deforestation, 1990 – 2000, Rural Sociology, 71:685–712.

Keesing, F., Belden, L.K., Daszak, P., Dobson, A., Harvell, C.D., Holt, R.D., Hudson, P., Jolles, A., Jones, K.E., Mitchell, C.E., Myers, S.S., Bogich, T., Ostfeld, R.S., 2010, Impacts of biodiversity on the emergence and transmission of infectious diseases, Nature, 468:647652.

Killilea, M.E., Swei, A., Lane, R.S., Briggs, C.J., Ostfeld, R.S. (2008). Spatial dynamics of lyme disease: a review. Ecohealth, 5(2), 167–195.

Kunkel, B., 2017, The Capitalocene, London Review of Books, 39(5):22–28.

Lambin, E.F., Meyfroidt, P., 2011, Global land use change, economic globalization, and the looming land scarcity, Proc. Natl. Acad. Sci. USA, 108:346572.

Lapola, D.M., Martinelli, L.A., Peres, C.A., Ometto, J.P.H.B., Ferreira, M.E., et al., 2014, Pervasive transition of the Brazilian land-use system, Nature Climate Change, 4:27–35.

Lerner, A.M., Eakin, H., 2011, An obsolete dichotomy? Rethinking the rural-urban interface in terms of food security and production in the global south, The Geographical Journal, 177(4):311320.

Liu, J., Dietz, T., Carpenter, S.R., Alberti, M., Folke, C., Moran, E., Pell, A.N., Deadman, P., Kratz, T., Lubchenco, J., Ostrom, E., Ouyang, Z., Provencher, W., Redman, C.L., Schneider, S.H., Taylor, W.W., 2007, Complexity of coupled human and natural systems, Science, 317(5844):1513–1516.

Lugo, A.E., 2009, The emerging era of novel tropical forests, Biotropica, 41, 589591.

Macdonald, G., 1957, The Epidemiology and Control of Malaria, Oxford University Press, London.

Mandal, S., Sakar, R., Sinha, S., 2011, Mathematical models of malaria – a review, Malaria Journal, 10/1/202 (online open access).

Mansfield, B., Munroe, D.K., McSweeny, K., 2010, Does economic growth cause environmental recovery? Geographical explanations of forest regrowth, Geography Compass, 4: 41627.

Mao, X., 2007, Stochastic Differential Equations and Applications, Harwood Publishing, Chichester UK.

Mao, X., 2007, Stochastic Differential Equations and Applications, Second Edition, Woodhead Publishing, Philadelphia.

McGarth, S., 2013, Fuelling global production networks with *slave labour*?: Migrant sugar cane workers in the Brazilian ethanol GPN. Geoforum, 44:32–43.

Mena I, Nelson MI, Quezada-Monroy F, Dutta J, Cortes-Fernndez R, Lara-Puente JH, Castro-Peralta F, et al., 2016, Origins of the 2009 H1N1 influenza pandemic in swine in Mexico, Elife, 5, pii:e16777. doi: https://doi.org/10.7554/eLife.16777.

Meyfroidt, P., Carlson, K.M., Fagan, M.F., Gutiérrez-Vlez, V.H., Macedo, M.N., et al., 2014, Multiple pathways of commodity crop expansion in tropical forest landscapes, Environ. Res. Lett., 9:074012.

Mills, J.H., Waite, T.A., 2009, Economic prosperity, biodiversity conservation, and the environmental Kuznets curve, Ecological Economics, 68:20872095.

Moench, M., Gyawali, D., 2008, Desakota: Reinterpreting the Urban-Rural Continuum. Part II: A Final Report of the Desakota Research Group, Natural Environment Research Council, London. Available online at https://assets.publishing.service.gov.uk/media/57a08bc3ed915d3cfd000f14/Desakota-Part-II-A.pdf.

Moore, J.W., 2015, Capitalism in the Web of Life: Ecology and the Accumulation of Capital, Verso, New York.

Moran, P.A.P., 1953, The statistical analysis of the Canadian lynx cycle. II. Synchronization and meteorology, Australian Journal of Zoology, 1:291–298.

Mota, M.T., Terzian, A.C., Silva, M.L., Estofolete, C., Nogueira, M.L., 2016, Mosquito-transmitted viruses - the great Brazilian challenge, Braz J Microbiol., 47 Suppl 1:38–50.

Nelson, M.I., Viboud, C., Vincent, A.L., Culhane, M.R., Detmer, S.E., Wentworth, D.E., Rambaut, A., et al., 2015, Global migration of influenza A viruses in swine, Nature Communications, 6:6696. doi: https://doi.org/10.1038/ncomms7696.

Noureddine, R., Chauvin, A., Plantard, O., 2011, Lack of genetic structure among Eurasian populations of the tick *Ixodes ricinus* contrasts with marked divergence from north-African populations, Int J Parasitol., 41(2):183–192.

Oliveira, G.L.T., 2016, The geopolitics of Brazilian soybeans, The Journal of Peasant Studies, 43(2):348–372.

Ostfeld, R.S., Canham, C.D., Oggenfuss, K., Winchcombe, R.J., Keesing, F., 2006, Climate, deer, rodents, and acorns as determinants of variation in Lyme-disease risk, PLoS Biol, 4(6):e145.

Pacheco, P., Poccard-Chapuis, R., 2012, The complex evolution of cattle ranching development amid market integration and policy shifts in the Brazilian Amazon, Annals of the Association of American Geographers, 102(6):1366–1390.

Padoch, C., Brondizio, E., Costa, S., Pinedo-Vasquez, M., Sears, R.R., Siqueira, A., 2008, Urban forest and rural cities: multi-sited households, consumption patterns, and forest resources in Amazonia, Ecology and Society, 13(2):2. Available online at http://www.ecologyandsociety. org/vol13/iss2/art2/.

Patel, R., 2013, The Long Green Revolution, The Journal of Peasant Studies, 40(1):1–63.

Perfecto, I., Vandermeer, J., 2010, The agroecological matrix as alternative to the land-sparing/ agriculture intensification model, Proc Natl Acad Sci U S A, 107(13):57865791.

Pham, T.T., Meng, S., Sun, Y., Lv, W., Bahl, J., 2016, Inference of Japanese encephalitis virus ecological and evolutionary dynamics from passive and active virus surveillance, Virus Evol. 2(1):vew009.

Predescu, M., Sirbu, G., Levins, R., Awerbuch-Friedlander, T., 2007, On the dynamics of a deterministic and stochastic model for mosquito control, Applied Mathematics Letters, 20(8):919–925.

Pyle, G.F., 1969, Diffusion of cholera in the United States, Geographical Analysis, 1:59–75.

Pyle, G.F., 1979, Applied Medical Geography, John Wiley Sons, New Jersey.

Raghavan, R.K., Goodin, D.G., Dryden, M.W., Hroobi, A., Gordon, D.M., Cheng, C., Nair, A.D., Jakkula, L.U., Hanzlicek, G.A., Anderson, G.A., Ganta, R.R., 2016, Heterogeneous associations of ecological attributes with tick-borne rickettsial pathogens in a periurban landscape, Vector Borne Zoonotic Dis., 16(9):569–576.

Raghavan, R.K., Neises, D., Goodin, D.G., Andresen, D.A., Ganta, R.R., 2014, Bayesian spatio-temporal analysis and geospatial risk factors of Human Monocytic Ehrlichiosis, PLoS ONE, 9(7):e100850.

Rede Social de Justiça e Direitos Humanos, GRAIN, Inter Pares, Solidarity Sweden – Latin America, 2015, *Foreign Pension Funds and Land Grabbing in Brazil*. Final report. Available online at https://www.grain.org/article/entries/5336-foreign-pension-funds-and-land-grabbing-in-brazil.pdf.

Reiner, R.C. Jr, Perkins, T.A., Barker, C.M., Niu, T., Chaves, L.F., Ellis, A.M., George, D.B., et al., 2013, A systematic review of mathematical models of mosquito-borne pathogen transmission: 1970-2010, J R Soc Interface., 10(81):20120921.

Reluga, T.C., 2016, The importance of being atomic: Ecological invasions as random walks instead of waves. Theor Popul Biol., 112:157–169.

Rezza, G., 2014, Dengue and chikungunya: long-distance spread and outbreaks in naïve areas, Pathog Glob Health, 108(8):349–355.

Robertson, C., Pant, D.P., Joshi, D.D., Sharma, M., Dahal, M., Stephen, C., 2013, Comparative spatial dynamics of Japanese Encephalitis and Acute Encephalitis Syndrome in Nepal, PLoS One, 8(7):e66168.

Rodriguez, D.J., Torres-Sorando, L., 2001, Models of infectious diseases in spatially heterogeneous environments, Bull. Math. Biol., 63:547–571. doi: https://doi.org/10.1006/bulm.2001.0231

Rosa, I., Souza, C., Ewers, R.M., 2012, Changes in size of deforested patches in the Brazilian Amazon, Conserv. Biol., 26:9327.

Rosenstock, T.S., Hastings, A., Koenig, W.D., Lyles, W.D., Brown, P.H., 2011, Testing Moran's theorem in an agrosystem, Okios, 120(9):1434–1440.

Ross, R., 1911, The Prevention of Malaria, Second Edition, Murray, London.

Salkeld, D.J., Nieto, N.C., Carbajales-Dale, P., Carbajales-Dale, M., Cinkovich, S.S., Lambin, E.F., 2015, Disease risk and landscape attributes of tick-borne Borrelia pathogens in the San Francisco Bay Area, California, PLoS ONE, 10(8):e0134812.

Samson, D.M., Archer, R.S., Alimi, T.O., Arheart, K.K., Impoinvil, D.E., Oscar, R., Fuller, D.O., Qualls, W.A., 2015, New baseline environmental assessment of mosquito ecology in northern Haiti during increased urbanization, J Vector Ecol., 40(1):4658.

Santos-Vega, M., Martinez, P.P., Pascual, M., 2016, Climate forcing and infectious disease transmission in urban landscapes: integrating demographic and socioeconomic heterogeneity, Annals of the New York Academy of Sciences, 1382:44–55.

Schmink, M., 1994, In L. Arizpe, M.P. Stone, D.C. Major (eds), Population and Environment: Rethinking the Debate, Westview, Bolder, CO, pp 253275.

Simões, M., Telo da Gama, M.M., Nunes, A., 2008, Stochastic fluctuations in epidemics on networks, J R Soc Interface, 5(22):555–566.

Tatem, A.J., Huang, Z., Das, A., Qi, Q., Roth, J., Qiu, Y., 2012, Air travel and vector-borne disease movement, Parasitology, 139(14):1816–1830.

Taylor, P.J., García Barrios, R., 1999, The dynamics of socio-environmental change and the limits of Neo-Malthusian environmentalism, In T. Mount, H. Shue, M. Dore (eds) Global Environmental Economics: Equity and the Limits to Markets, Blackwell, Oxford, UK.

Torres-Sorando, L., Rodriguez, D.J., 1997, Models of spatio-temporal dynamics in malaria, Ecological Modelling, 104:231–240.

Turzi, M. 2011, The soybean republic, Yale Journal of International Affairs, 6(2):5968.

Wallace, D., 2017a, personal communication.

Wallace, R., 2017b, Information Theory Models of Instabilities in Critical Systems, World Scientific, Singapore.

Wallace, R., Wallace, D., Andrews, H., 1997, AIDS, tuberculosis, violent crime and low birthweight in eight US metropolitan regions, Environment and Planning A, 29:525–555.

Wallace, R., Ullmann, J., Wallace, D., Andrews, H., 1999, Deindustrialization, inner city decay, and the hierarchical diffusion of AIDS in the US, Environment and Planning A, 31:113–139.

Wallace, R.G., 2012, Beware the blob, Farming Pathogens blog, 30 November. Available online at https://farmingpathogens.wordpress.com/2012/11/30/beware-the-blob/.

Wallace, R.G., 2016a, Big Farms Make Big Flu: Dispatches on Infectious Disease, Agribusiness, and the Nature of Science. Monthly Review Press, New York.

Wallace, R.G., 2016b, Strange cotton, In Big Farms Make Big Flu: Dispatches on Infectious Diseases, Agribusiness, and the Nature of Science, Monthly Review Press, New York.

Wallace, R.G., Bergmann, L., Kock, R., Gilbert, M., Hogerwerf, L., Wallace, R., Holmberg, M., 2015, The dawn of Structural One Health: A new science tracking disease emergence along circuits of capital, Social Science and Medicine, 129:68–77.

Wallace, R.G., Kock, R.A., 2012, Whose food footprint? Capitalism, agriculture and the environment, Human Geography, 5(1):6383.

Wallace, R.G., Wallace, R., 2003, The geographic search engine: one way urban epidemics find susceptible populations and evade public health intervention. Journal of Urban Health, 80(S2):ii15. Abstract 03298, Second International Urban Health Conference, New York City.

Wallace, R.G., Wallace, R. (eds.), 2016, Neoliberal Ebola: Modeling Disease Emergence from Finance to Forest and Farm, Springer, Switzerland.

Walter, J.A., Sheppard, L.W., Anderson, T.L., Kastens, J.H., Bjrnstad, O.N. Liebhold, A.M., Reuman, D.C., 2017, The geography of spatial synchrony, Ecology Letters, 20(7):801–814.

Walter, K.S., Pepin, K.M., Webb, C.T., Gaff, H.D., Krause, P.J., Pitzer, V.E., Diuk-Wasser, M.A., 2016, Invasion of two tick-borne diseases across New England: harnessing human surveillance data to capture underlying ecological invasion processes, Proc Biol Sci., 283(1832). pii: 20160834.

Wright, A.L., Wolford, W., 2003, To Inherit the Earth: The Landless Movement and the Struggle for a New Brazil, Food First Books, Oakland, CA.

Yang, H., Ferreira, M., 2000, Assessing the effects of global warming and local social and economic conditions on the malaria transmission, Revista de Saude Publica, 34:214–222.

Yang, H., 2000, Malaria transmission model for different levels of acquired immunity and temperature-dependent parameters (vector), Revista de Saude Publica, 34:223–231.

Zhang, Q., Sun, K., Chinazzi, M., Pastore, Y., Piontti, A., Dean, N.E., Rojas, D.P., et al., 2017, Spread of Zika virus in the Americas, Proceedings of the National Academy of Sciences U S A. pii: 201620161. doi: https://doi.org/10.1073/pnas.1620161114. [Epub ahead of print]

Zhu, G., Liu, J., Tan, Q., Shi, B., 2016, Inferring the spatio-temporal patterns of dengue transmission from surveillance data in Guangzhou, China, PLoS Negl Trop Dis., 10(4):e0004633.

Chapter 3
Modeling State Interventions

3.1 A Control Theory Model of Disease Control

In the context of the modern nation state, the ecology of infectious diseases cannot be described by interacting populations alone, as much of the modeling literature implicitly presumes (Wallace and Wallace 2016). Modern states incorporate elaborate public health bureaucracies tasked with either containing or eliminating pathogen outbreaks. States are thus highly cognitive entities at the institutional level. It is then appropriate, indeed arguably necessary, to reconsider vector-borne infection from a control theory perspective.

Cognition, following the model of Atlan and Cohen (1998), involves choosing one of many possible responses to a stimulus. Choice reduces uncertainty in a formal manner, a reduction that implies the existence of an information source (Wallace 2015, 2017).

We assume that the underlying two-dimensional disease ecosystem is in explosive mode, i.e., either sudden ecosystem "smoothing" has occurred or a change in socioeconomic policy has imposed cross-effect noise, as in Fig. 2.4 or Eqs. (2.9) and (2.10). Thus the system becomes unstable, and corrective policy must be chosen and imposed, implying not only "control information" exists but that it is effective.

We enter the realm where information and control theories intersect. More precisely, the data rate theorem (DRT) (Nair et al. 2007) establishes the minimum rate at which externally supplied control information must be provided for an inherently unstable system to maintain stability. The first approximation assumes a linear expansion near a nonequilibrium steady state, in which actors of a dynamic system produce each other at a constant distribution. An n-dimensional vector of system parameters at time t, say xt, determines the state at time $t + 1$ according to the model of Fig. 3.1 as

© Springer International Publishing AG 2018
R. Wallace et al., *Clear-Cutting Disease Control*,
https://doi.org/10.1007/978-3-319-72850-6_3

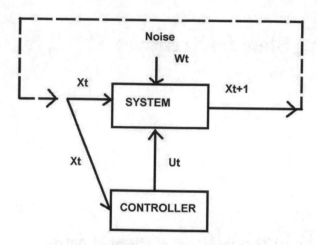

Fig. 3.1 A linear expansion near a nonequilibrium steady state of an inherently unstable control system, for which $x_{t+1} = \mathbf{A}x_t + \mathbf{B}u_t + W_t$. $\mathbf{A}$, $\mathbf{B}$ are square matrices, x_t the vector of system parameters at time t, u_t the control vector at time t, and W_t a white noise vector. The data rate theorem states that the minimum rate at which control information must be provided for system stability is $H > \log[|\det[\mathbf{A}^m]|]$, where $\mathbf{A}^m$ is the subcomponent of $\mathbf{A}$ having eigenvalues ≥ 1. This is interpreted as asserting that the rate of control information must exceed the rate at which the unstable system generates topological information

$$x_{t+1} = \mathbf{A}x_t + \mathbf{B}u_t + W_t \tag{3.1}$$

$\mathbf{A}$ and $\mathbf{B}$ are fixed $n \times n$ matrices, u_t is the vector of control information, and W_t is an n-dimensional vector of white noise. The data rate theorem under such conditions states that the minimum control information rate H necessary for system stability is determined by the relation

$$H > \log[|\det\left[\mathbf{A}^m\right]|] \equiv a_0 \tag{3.2}$$

where, for $m \leq n$, $\mathbf{A}_m$ is the subcomponent of $\mathbf{A}$ having eigenvalues ≥ 1. The right-hand side of Eq. (3.2) is interpreted as the rate at which the system generates "topological information."

The essence of the DRT is the onset of instability if the inequality of Eq. (3.2) is violated. Here we will use the rate distortion theorem (RDT) in conjunction with the stochastic self-stabilization theorem to examine in more detail the dynamics leading to control failure under increasing noise.

We examine the manner in which a control signal u_t emitted by the control source producing information at the rate H at time t is expressed in the system response x_{t+1}. Assume it is possible to deterministically retranslate an observed sequence of system outputs $X^i = x_1^i, x_2^i, \ldots$ into a sequence of possible control signals that is written as $\hat{U}^i = \hat{u}_0^i, \hat{u}_1^i, \ldots$, and compare that sequence with the original control sequence $U^i = u_0^i, u_1^i, \ldots$. The difference between them has a particular value under some chosen distortion measure:

$$d\left(z^n, \hat{z}^n\right) = \frac{1}{n}\sum_{i=1}^{n} d\left(z_i, \hat{z}_i\right) \tag{3.3}$$

so that the distortion for a sequence is the average of the per symbol distortion of the elements of the sequence. (See Cover and Thomas (2006) for details.)

An average distortion can then be defined as

$$D = \sum_{j} p\left(U^j\right) d\left(U^j, \hat{U}^j\right) \tag{3.4}$$

where $p(U^i)$ is the probability of the sequence U^i and $d(U^i, \hat{U}^i)$ is the distortion between U^i and the sequence of control signals that has been deterministically reconstructed from the system output.

According to the rate distortion theorem, for certain classes of channels, there exists a rate distortion function, $R(D)$, that determines the minimum channel capacity necessary to keep the average distortion below some fixed real number limit $D \geq 0$. Based on Feynman's (2000) interpretation of information as a form of free energy, it becomes possible to construct a Boltzmann-like pseudo-probability in the "temperature" of the control information rate H as

$$dP\left(R, \kappa, H\right) = \frac{\exp\left[-R/\kappa H\right] dR}{\int_0^\infty \exp\left[-R/\kappa H\right] dR} \tag{3.5}$$

where the dimensionless quantity κ parameterizes the degree to which the control signal produced at the rate H is actually effective. Higher values of κH must necessarily be associated with greater system channel capacity and hence less distortion between what the control instructs and the actual system response.

The denominator can be interpreted as a statistical mechanical partition function, and it becomes possible to define a "free energy" Morse function (Pettini 2007) F as

$$\exp\left[-F/\kappa H\right] \equiv \int_0^\infty \exp\left[-R/\kappa H\right] dR = \kappa H \tag{3.6}$$

so that $F(\kappa H) = -\kappa H \log[\kappa H]$.

See Chap. 5 for an introduction to Morse theory.

Then, assuming H is fixed, an "entropy" can be defined as the Legendre transform of F in κ,

$$S = F\left(\kappa\right) - \kappa \partial F / \partial \kappa = \kappa H \tag{3.7}$$

The Onsager approximation of nonequilibrium thermodynamics (de Groot and Mazur 1984) can now be invoked, based on the gradient of S in κ at the fixed rate of control information H so that a stochastic Onsager equation can be written describing the dynamics of κ as

$$d\kappa_t = \mu \partial S / \partial \kappa \, dt + \sigma g(\kappa_t) dW_t = \mu H dt + \sigma g(\kappa_t) dW_t \tag{3.8}$$

μ is a coefficient indexing the attempt by the system – here, the modern state – to penetrate the inevitable "fog-of-war" confusion surrounding, in this case, regulation during normal times and intervention during an emergency. The second term, in σ $g(\kappa_t)$, is a white noise volatility measure, representing the density of that fog. Recall that larger κH will be associated with higher R and hence smaller distortion between intent and effect.

We have reduced the two-dimensional vector-borne pandemic to a one-dimensional control theory problem that falls under an inversion of the simplest version of the stochastic stabilization theorem, i.e., sufficiently large system "noise" σ can drive κ to zero, a converse of the previous argument, as small κH will violate the strictures of the DRT, releasing the pandemic outbreak.

The appearance of the log term in Eq. (3.2) suggests the possibility of a nuanced — if heuristic — approach that applies the Itô chain rule to $\log[\kappa]$ using Eq. (3.8), providing a more detailed picture of system failure. Since the log is a concave function, Jensen's inequality (Cover and Thomas 2006) implies that, in terms of the expectation E, we again have

$$\log\left[E(x)\right] \geq E\left(\log[x]\right) \tag{3.9}$$

so the procedure produces a lower limit for the expectation of κ, remembering that sufficient noise 'tests the limit', driving it essentially to zero.

We assume $g(\kappa) = \sqrt{\kappa^2 + \alpha^2}$ in Eq. (3.8), so that there is residual volatility even for small κ. This produces the stochastic differential equation:

$$d\kappa_t = \mu H dt + \sigma \sqrt{\kappa^2 + \alpha^2} \, dW_t \tag{3.10}$$

Expanding $\log[\kappa_t]$ using the Itô chain rule gives a relation

$$d\kappa(t) / dt = \mu H - \frac{1}{2}\kappa(t)\sigma^2 - \frac{1}{2}\frac{\sigma^2 \alpha^2}{\kappa(t)} \tag{3.11}$$

where the terms in σ represent the typical Itô correction factor. Recall that $d \log(x)/dt = (1/x)dx/dt$. We are, then, calculating the dynamics of $E(\log[\kappa])$ and making a heuristic application of Jensen's inequality to estimate a lower limit on $E(\kappa)$.

There are two nonequilibrium steady-state (nss) solutions characterizing lower-limit dynamics. Some exploration using the DEploy tool of the computer algebra system Maple shows the larger solution is stable but declines with increasing σ. The smaller solution increases monotonically with σ but is not stable, either collapsing to zero or rising to the larger NSS. The expectations satisfy inequalities

$$E\left(\kappa_{La}\right) \geq \frac{\mu H + \sqrt{H^2 \mu^2 - \alpha^2 \sigma^2}}{\sigma^2}$$
$$E\left(\kappa_{Sm}\right) \geq \frac{\mu H - \sqrt{H^2 \mu^2 - \alpha^2 \sigma^2}}{\sigma^2} \tag{3.12}$$

This result represents a parsing of stability conditions beyond the stochastic stability theorem. However, if $H\mu < \alpha\sigma^2$, the two branches coalesce, and no stability is possible. Thus we recover a further necessary condition for stability as

$$H > \frac{\alpha\sigma^2}{\mu} \tag{3.13}$$

Violation of this condition drives the "effectiveness" parameter κ to zero, suggesting, in the next section, another iteration of the data rate theorem.

3.2 A Cognitive Model of Disease Control

The data rate theorem argument we presented in the previous section suggests a greater probability that a stabilized pathogen system will transition to unstable behavior if the temperature analog κH falls below a critical value.

We can extend the perspective to more complicated patterns of phase transition via the "cognitive paradigm" of Atlan and Cohen (1998), under which a system, such as the modern nation state exercising public health power, is considered cognitive if it compares incoming signals with a learned or inherited picture of the world, then actively chooses a response from a larger set. Choice, as we described in the previous section, implies the existence of an information source, as it reduces uncertainty in a formal way (Wallace 2015, 2017).

In the section above, we introduced the notion government public health policy engages in such group cognition. Given such a "dual" information source – government vs disease – associated with such an inherently unstable cognitive system of interest, an equivalence class algebra can be constructed by choosing different system origin states and defining the equivalence of subsequent states at a later time by the existence of a high-probability path connecting them to the same origin state.

Disjoint partition by equivalence class, analogous to orbit equivalence classes in dynamical systems, defines a symmetry groupoid associated with the cognitive process (Wallace 2015, 2017). Groupoids are generalizations of group symmetries in which there is not necessarily a product defined for each possible element pair (Weinstein 1996). An example would be the disjoint union of different groups.

See Chap. 5 for an introduction to groupoid theory.

Nation states are comprised of functional nodes – different agencies, different competing interests – which must connect and collaborate to solve a societal problem or remain disconnected and fail to act (Chappell 2018). How the nodes connect determines whether group cognition can be turned onto a public health problem.

The equivalence classes across possible origin states define a set of information sources dual to different cognitive states available to the inherently unstable cognitive system. These create a large groupoid, with each orbit corresponding to a transitive groupoid, whose disjoint union is the full groupoid. Each subgroupoid is associated with its own dual information source, and larger groupoids must have richer dual information sources than smaller.

Let X_{G_i} be the system's dual information source associated with groupoid element G_i. We next construct a Morse function (Pettini 2007) in a standard manner, using $T \equiv \kappa H$ as a temperature analog.

Let $H\left(X_{G_i}\right) \equiv H_{G_i}$ be the Shannon uncertainty of the information source associated with the groupoid element G_i. Define another Boltzmann-like pseudo-probability as

$$P\left[H_{G_i}\right] \equiv \frac{\exp\left[-H_{G_i}/T\right]}{\sum_j \exp\left[-H_{G_i}/T\right]} \tag{3.14}$$

where the sum is over the different possible cognitive modes of the full system.

Another "free-energy" Morse function F can then be defined as

$$\exp\left[-F/T\right] \equiv \sum_j \exp\left[-H_{G_i}/T\right]$$

$$F = -T \log\left[\sum_j \exp\left[-H_{G_i}/T\right]\right] \tag{3.15}$$

As a consequence of the underlying groupoid-generalized symmetries associated with high-order cognition, as opposed to simple control theory, it is possible to apply an extension of Landau's version of phase transition (Pettini 2007). Landau argued that spontaneous symmetry breaking of a group structure represents phase change in physical systems, with the higher energies available at higher temperatures being more symmetric. The shift between symmetries is highly punctuated in the "temperature" index $T = \kappa H$ – but in the context of groupoid rather than group symmetries.

Based on the analogy with physical systems, there should be only a few possible phases, with highly punctuated transitions between them as the fog-of-war "temperature" T decreases, either as the effects of "friction" become manifest, decreasing κ, or by decline in the rate of control information H.

For nonergodic systems the groupoids become trivial, associated with the individual high-probability paths for which an H-value may be defined, although that cannot be represented in the form of a Shannon "entropy" (Khinchin 1957, p. 72).

The policy implications orbit about the institutional control parameter κH. Minimal erosion in the parameter – a variance in regulation here, a corrupt blind eye there, tolerating some minor intimidation of local dissent or an outright campaign of murdering environmental activists (Global Witness 2014) – can trigger a very sudden collapse in disease control. Under such a regime, enforcement efforts, once the disease carrier – here a mosquito population – has escaped, need to be ramped up to an extreme level just to get atop a spreading outbreak that has broken across thresholds in populations infected and geographic space. Such punctuated dynamics may well involve considerable hysteresis, the complication of long-trailing effects across the system, once initial barriers to infection fall.

The implication here is that good governance, protected agricultural commons, farmer autonomy, conservation agroecology, urban public health, community resilience, and biocontrol are foundationally integrated (Hanspach et al. 2017; Rotz and Fraser 2015; Wallace et al. 2018).

3.3 A Ratchet Mechanism

Disease outbreaks are rarely about the pathogen or clinical outcomes alone in cause or effect. An outbreak can drive the very conditions that brought about its initial emergence into a new phase or degrade a government's capacity to respond.

Recall the derivation of Eq. (3.6), in terms of the rate distortion function of the channel connecting the controller with the system under control:

$$\exp\left[-F / \kappa H\right] = \int_{0}^{\infty} \exp\left[-R / \kappa H\right] dR = \kappa H \equiv T \tag{3.16}$$

We suppose that T is fixed, but $T \to T + \Delta, 0 \leq \Delta \ll T$. Thus

$$\exp\left[-F / (T + \Delta)\right] = T + \Delta \tag{3.17}$$

and we can define a new "entropy" as $S = F(\Delta) - \Delta \, \partial F / \partial \Delta$ leading to the stochastic differential equation:

$$d\Delta_t = \frac{\mu \Delta_t}{T + \Delta_t} dt + \sigma \Delta_t dW_t \approx \frac{\mu}{T} \Delta_t dt + \sigma \Delta_t dW_t \tag{3.18}$$

where μ is a new 'diffusion coefficient' and σ a new 'noise' parameter and dW_t represents the usual white noise, and we have used the condition that $0 \leq \Delta \ll T$.

Applying the stochastic stabilization theorem,

$$\lim_{t \to \infty} \frac{\log\left[|\Delta_t|\right]}{t} \to < 0 \tag{3.19}$$

unless

$$\mu/T > \frac{1}{2}\sigma^2$$
$$T < \frac{2\mu}{\sigma^2} \tag{3.20}$$

This places an upper limit on $T = \kappa H$. More importantly, it establishes the possibility of a public health analog to an economic ratchet.

Suppose "structural adjustment" or other neoliberal policy triggers a reduction in the ability of a polity to implement public health measures, so that T declines in the face of endemic or episodic disease. The resulting rise in disease prevalence and incidence then causes social disintegration that increases σ so that the disease outbreak itself interferes with the ability to carry out needed public health interventions. T then declines even further, σ rises again, the outbreak becomes more severe, and a race to the bottom ensues. Hemorrhagic fevers, SARS, and MERS-CoV offer classic nosocomial examples, but such ratchets can extend beyond the hospital setting and across the social fabric, from mosquito control to the very function of the state (Ho et al. 2003; De Waal 2003; Fisher-Hoch 2005; Whiteford and Hill 2005; Shin et al. 2017).

3.4   Effectiveness, Efficiency, and Their Synergism

The argument above can be made more precise by abducting an approach from the Arrhenius treatment of reaction rates, where the rate at which resources are provided is the temperature analog. Using this method we can examine the classic conflict between efficiency and effectiveness so often commented on in the management science literature. In addition, we can study their synergistic interaction.

"Public health" is the result of collaboration across a number of institutional entities in the control theory sense leading to Eqs. (3.5) and (3.6), indexed as $j = 1...n$. Each entity consumes resources at some rate M_j under an overall constraint $M - \sum_j M_j = 0$, and we are interested in the response rate of each entity, above some "action trigger threshold." For such entities the response rate will be proportional to the probability that the channel rate distortion function connecting entity to outcome is greater than some "action threshold" R_j^0:

$$P\left[R_j \geq R_j^0\right] = \frac{\int_{R_j^0}^{\infty} \exp\left[-R_j / M_j\right] dR_j}{\int_0^{\infty} \exp\left[-R_j / M_j\right] dR_j} = \exp\left[-R_j^0 / M_j\right] \tag{3.21}$$

The effectiveness and efficiency of a particular entity can then be expressed as the two quantities

$$\exp\left[-R_j^0 / M_j\right]$$
$$\frac{\exp\left[-R_j^0 / M_j\right]}{M_j} \tag{3.22}$$

Short-term goals in public health surround effectiveness, while long-term plans are confronted with the need to maximize efficiency, i.e., the expression $\sum_j \exp\left[-R_j^0 / M_j\right] / M_j$ under the overall constraint on resources provided to public health measures, $M - \sum_j M_j = 0$.

Paying dues to the economists, we first examine efficiency.

Let

$$L \equiv \sum_j \frac{\exp\left[-R_j^0 / M_j\right]}{M_j} + \lambda\left(M - \sum_j M_j\right) \tag{3.23}$$

where λ is the Lagrange undetermined multiplier.

The gradient equations determining the maximum of efficiency under the resource constraint are then

$$\frac{R_j^0 \exp\left[-R_j^0 / M_j\right]}{M_j^3} - \frac{\exp\left[-R_j^0 / M_j\right]}{M_j^2} = \lambda$$

$$M = \sum_j M_j \tag{3.24}$$

$$\partial L / \partial M = \lambda$$

where, abducting arguments from physical theory, λ is taken as an inverse response temperature. Figure 3.2 shows a single term for $R_j^0 = 0.5$ over the range $0 \leq M \leq 1$.

It is easy to show that $\lambda = 0$ for $M_j = R_j^0$.

For negative response temperature, i.e., $\partial L/\partial M = \lambda < 0$, the individual M_j can become unconstrained, closely analogous to the excited state of a "pumped" physical system like a laser. As a consequence, if the disease outbreak "gets inside the command decision loop" of the bureaucratic entities constituting the "public health" response, so that λ becomes negative, then resource demands cannot be met under

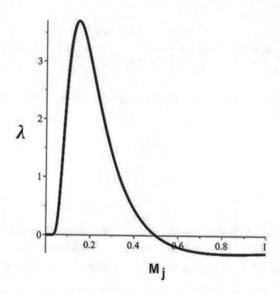

Fig. 3.2 Optimization relation of the second term of Eq. (3.24) for a single module with $R_0 = 0.5$. For positive response temperature, $\lambda > 0$, the M_j is constrained and the condition $M = \sum_j M_j$ can be met. For negative response temperature, the M_j can become unconstrained, like the excited state of a "pumped" physical system, for example, a laser. If the disease outbreak "gets inside the command decision loop" of the bureaucratic entities constituting the "public health" response, so that $\lambda < 0$, then resource demands cannot be met under the constraint relation, and the infection outbreak proliferates until it burns out

the constraint relation, and the infection outbreak will proliferate until it burns out or becomes high-level endemic.

Efficiency is only one aspect of public health intervention. In the face of a spreading pandemic with high morbidity and mortality, effectiveness becomes paramount. Then we must optimize

$$L = \sum_j \exp\left[-R_j^0 / M_j\right] - \lambda \left[\sum_j M_j - M\right] \tag{3.25}$$

leading to the relation $R_j^0 \exp[-R_j^0 / M_j / M_j^2] = \lambda$ as shown in Fig. 3.3. Here, λ is never negative, but small values imply unconstrained demand for resource M_j, an impossible condition.

Again, while Fig. 3.2 may apply to long-time strategic time scales, Fig. 3.3 is more appropriate to tactical "do-or-die" time frames.

More generally, strategy, the long-time frame, and tactics, the immediate challenges, will become synergistic, leading to optimization of the product term:

$$\frac{\exp\left[-R_j^0 / M_j\right]\exp\left[-R_j^0 / M_j\right]}{M_j} - \frac{\exp\left[-2R_j^0 / M_j\right]}{M_j} \tag{3.26}$$

Fig. 3.3 Direct optimization of response rate, without concern for long-term efficiency. Again, $K = 0.5$. No negative temperature "pumped" states exist, but small values of λ imply tactical resource demands that simply cannot be met

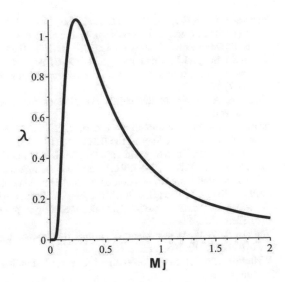

This gives a functional form exactly like Fig. 3.2 but with the node $\lambda = 0$ at $2R_j^0$ instead of R_j^0.

The implication, at both tactical and strategic scales, is that sufficient "structural adjustment" or unconstrained agroecological exploitation in the face of stagnant "public health" resources can allow disease outbreaks to proceed more rapidly than a weakened state bureaucracy can respond. It appears an obvious point often lost: diseases are more than objects on which we act. Some are capable of degrading the very public health capacity they attract.

References

Atlan, H., Cohen, I., 1998, Immune information, self-organization and meaning, International Immunology, 10:711–717.

Chappell, M.J., 2018, Beginning to End Hunger: Food and the Environment in Belo Horizonte, Brazil, and Beyond, University of California Press, Berkeley.

Cover, T., Thomas, J., 2006, Elements of Information Theory, Second Edition, Wiley, New York.

de Groot, S., P. Mazur, 1984, Non-Equilibrium Thermodynamics, Dover, New York.

De Waal, A., 2003, How will HIV/AIDS transform African governance?, African Affairs, 102:1–23.

Feynman, R., 2000, Lectures in Computation, Westview Press, Boulder, CO.

Fisher-Hoch, S.P., 2005, Lessons from nosocomial viral haemorrhagic fever outbreaks, Br Med Bull., 73-74:123–137.

Global Witness, 2014, Deadly Environment: The Dramatic Rise in Killings of Environmental and Land Defenders. London, UK. Available online at https://www.globalwitness.org/en/campaigns/environmental-activists/deadly-environment/.

Hanspach, J., Abson, D.J., French Collier, N.F., Dorrestijn, I., Schultner, J., Fischer, J., 2017, From trade-offs to synergies in food security and biodiversity conservation, Frontiers in Ecology and the Environment. doi: https://doi.org/10.1002/fee.1632.

Ho, A.S., Sung, J.J., Chan-Yeung, M., 2003, An outbreak of severe acute respiratory syndrome among hospital workers in a community hospital in Hong Kong, Ann Intern Med., 139(7):564–567.

Khinchin, A., 1957, Mathematical Foundations of Information Theory, Dover Publications, New York.

Nair, G., Fagnani, F., Zampieri, S., Evans, R., 2007, Feedback control under data rate constraints: an overview, Proceedings of the IEEEE, 95:108–137.

Pettini, M., 2007, Geometry and Topology in Hamiltonian Dynamics, Springer, New York.

Rotz, S., Fraser, E.D.G., 2015, Resilience and the industrial food system: analyzing the impacts of agricultural industrialization on food system vulnerability, J Environ Stud Sci, 5:459–473

Shin, N., Kwag, T., Park, S., Kim, Y.H., 2017, Effects of operational decisions on the diffusion of epidemic disease: A system dynamics modeling of the MERS-CoV outbreak in South Korea, J Theor Biol. 421:39–50.

Wallace, R., 2015, An Information Approach to Mitochondrial Dysfunction: Extending Swerdlow's hypothesis, World Scientific, Singapore.

Wallace, R., 2017, Information Theory Models of Instabilities in Critical Systems, World Scientific, Singapore.

Wallace, R.G., Alders, R., Kock, R., Jonas, T., Wallace, R., Hogerwerf, L., 2018, Health before medicine: Community resilience in food landscapes, In M. Walton (ed.), One Planet - Eco-One Health: Looking After Humans, Animals and the Environment, Sydney University Press, Sydney.

Wallace, R.G., Wallace, R. (eds.), 2016, Neoliberal Ebola: Modeling Disease Emergence from Finance to Forest and Farm, Springer, Switzerland.

Weinstein, A., 1996, Groupoids: unifying internal and external symmetry, Notices of the American Mathematical Association, 43:744–752.

Whiteford, L., Hill, B., 2005, The political ecology of dengue in Cuba and the Dominican Republic, In G. Guest (ed), Globalization, Health, and the Environment: An Integrated Perspective, AltaMira Press, Lanham, MD, pp. 219–237.

Chapter 4
Implications for Disease Intervention and Modeling

Check for updates

4.1 A Political History of Vector-Borne Infection

The epidemiological fates of novel and long-circulating diseases depend on their context, a causality found in the field as much as in the object (Dobson and Carper 1996; Wolfe et al. 2007; Wallace 2016a, b; Jones et al. 2017).

In the formalism presented here, we described the manifold effects of environmental stochasticity as captured by a system of Itô stochastic differential equations imposed upon a vector-pathogen-host system, a context embodying the complexity and diversity of forest interactions and urban public health. Given a particular shift in the pattern of "noise," a pathogen population in such a system can become suddenly destabilized, with sequentially rising peaks a characteristic outcome. Following a modeling literature back to Ross (1911), the result implies that depending on its source — in this case, agroecological practice and urban policy — environmental noise can promote as much as retard pathogen population growth.

As a matter of principle, such a result is all well and good, but in terms of interventions by which a government might pursue, how exactly is this epidemiological noise embodied? Alongside "ecological" inputs, such as nonhuman vertebrate hosts, vector species competition, and geographic variation in vector competence, much attention has been paid to social and environmental factors, including climate change, urbanization, water storage practices, human migration and transportation, mosquito-proof housing, and insecticide resistance (Lindsay et al. 2002; Carlson et al. 2016; Tabachnick 2016; Ali et al. 2017; Shragai et al. 2017; Weber et al. 2017).

These are clearly important factors. At the same time, many are proximate and even consequentialist in bias, the latter associated with an outbreak only long after a pathogen emerges. Whatever their point of entry, the bulk of factors are themselves structured by the ostensible geological force into which capitalism, here specifically in its agroeconomic and urban manifestation, has developed (Foster et al. 2010; Moore 2015; Wallace et al. 2016; Muntaner and Wallace 2018; Wallace et al. 2018).

A government at the mercy of global capitalism may choose to intervene at the more proximate levels, as our control theory modeling here addresses, even if as much to save face as to protect its populace. Few epidemiologists would object to a decision to provide the expenditures necessary to drain standing pools of water in which mosquitoes breed in the cities. But what of the adjunct conundrum? International financial institutions routinely impose structural adjustment programs that in return for stopgap loans require defunding these very domestic public and animal health programs (Pfeiffer and Chapman 2010; Enticott et al. 2011; Amankwah et al. 2014; Wallace et al. 2015; Sparke 2016).

Pathogens rarely cooperate with such political economies. The webs of causality run across biocultural domains, including molecular, natural selection, agroecology, and circuits of capital driving development and deforestation. One can start an explanation for an outbreak at any point along these networks, whose modeling and variables inputted are fundamentally social decisions (Levins 1998). For vector-borne diseases, we can begin where many research groups focus. Vittor's group (2006, 2009), for instance, layers a variety of proximate socioecological inputs from agricultural source to urban sink, which Vittor (2016) summarizes:

> We found that deforestation followed by agriculture and regrowth of low-lying vegetation provided a much more suitable environment for the malaria mosquito carrier than pristine forest. Increasing urbanization and poverty create a fertile environment for the mosquitoes that spread dengue by creating ample breeding sites. In addition, climate change may raise the temperature and/or humidity in areas that previously have been below the threshold required for the mosquitoes to thrive... Urbanization, changing climate, air travel and transportation, and waxing and waning control efforts that are at the mercy of economic and political factors have led to these mosquitoes spreading to new areas and coming back in areas where they had previously been eradicated.

Much work has shown urbanized pockets of poverty, in conjunction with poor sanitation, poor drainage, and standing water, to be terrific breeding sites for mosquitoes (e.g., Caprara et al. 2009; Mota et al. 2016). Structural adjustment has degraded surveillance efforts and ended many a control effort, permitting mosquitoes freer range, especially the adaptable *Ae. aegypti*, which lays quiescent eggs, can oviposit in multiple places, and bites many times in a single gonotrophic cycle. A burgeoning literature imputes this "downstream" degradation as the neoliberal program operationalized (Nading 2014; Kelly and Lezaun 2014; Kentikelenis et al. 2014; Johnson 2017; Dzingirai et al. 2017).

It was by virtue of this shifting context that Weaver and Reisen (2010) predicted imminent spikes in arboviruses:

> Perhaps the greatest health risk of arboviral emergence comes from extensive tropical urbanization and the colonization of this expanding habitat by the highly anthropophilic (attracted to humans) mosquito, *Aedes aegypti*. These factors led to the emergence of perma- nent endemic cycles of urban DENV and chikungunya virus (CHIKV), as well as seasonal interhuman transmission of yellow fever and Zika viruses...

> There is reason to believe that additional viruses such as [Venezuelan equine encephalitis virus], [Zika virus] and [Mayaro virus] have the potential for urbanization, which could have devastating public health consequences, especially in the Western Hemisphere, where

there is no herd immunity. The movement of rural *Aedes* and *Culex* vectors and their hosts into urban and peridomestic environments allow effective amplification within simplified transmission cycles in close proximity to humans.

Weaver and Reisen placed the urbanization of the viruses and their vectors in its socioeconomic context:

> The tropical urbanization that has accelerated since World War II, combined with the multiple interhemispheric introductions of both *Ae. aegypti* and *Ae. albopictus*, has greatly increased the population densities and geographic ranges of these vectors. *Ae. aegypti* is especially aided by poverty when the lack of municipal water services results in intradomiciliary water storage and the lack of trash collection results in the accumulation of waste receptacles that hold rainwater to support larval development.

After more than a hundred years of social geographies of vector-borne diseases, the role poverty plays is at this point a veritable scientific law, even as the specifics differ place to place. In a summary of the literature, including Angelo Celli's (1900, 1925) seminal work, Chaves (2013) connects the spread of the latifundia model of land development to deforestation, epidemiological shocks, and back again to land expropriation:

> Deforestation has also been long recognized as one of the major drivers for the emergence of infectious diseases affecting humans, with studies documenting the emergence of malaria, leishmaniasis and yellow fever shortly after large scale land use changes. An additional insight from the study of the association between malaria emergence and deforestation was the correlation of malaria endemicity with the formation of latifundia, i.e., the accumulation of land tenure by a small number of landowners, a pattern observed both in the Agro-Pontino Romano for centuries, and Spain during the 1930s.

> More specifically, it has been suggested, and documented, by the long historical records for the Roman Agro-Pontino, that deforestation and agricultural development led to ideal conditions for the development of mosquito vectors of malaria parasites, a fact biologically instantiated by ecological research over recent years. The debilitating effects of malaria on farmers reduce their ability to harvest crops and lead to the sale or abandonment and adjudication of land by healthier and/or wealthier landowners that will underutilize land as latifundia, i.e., large states whose exploitation, because of the landmass size, require the labor of workers who do not own the land. When land cover is primarily forested, land tenure can be redistributed for agricultural exploitation, and in turn result in a repeated cycle of agricultural exploitation, malaria transmission and latifundia formation.

The latifundia model of social reproduction, and, as a growing literature indicates, its neoliberal analogs, can promote disease emergence, while, in the other direction, in a variation of the ratchet process modeled in the previous chapter, disease outbreaks can drive the very consolidation that selected for them. Chaves (2013) simulates the process by coupling a susceptible-infected-susceptible transmission model to a deterministic transition matrix across landowners and land parcels, concluding:

> Our simulations showed that two key elements of Celli's original hypothesis are, indeed, fundamental to the formation of latifundia: (i) the decreased utility of land exploitation by the reduced labor ability of sick landowners...and (ii) differences in the risk to acquire infections. In that sense our model can mechanistically confirm one of the main observations made by Celli, i.e., that people that were protected from disease transmission were more likely to either conserve and/or purchase land from people that were susceptible to disease transmission...

These results suggest that inequities in the protection against a disease, for example the use and access to disease prevention devices, can promote further socio-economic inequities in societies where a disease is endemically persistent or has frequent epidemics. This phenomenon has been observed in malaria, where inequities in access to insecticides treated nets can feed positive feedback loops further increasing socio-economic differences within a host population.

In essence, pathogens indirectly act as veritable bioeconomic weapons that initiate new rounds of land grabbing and wealth concentration, a highly unstable system of positive reinforcement. Ijumba and Lindsay (2001) propose such mechanisms may arise in part out of a "paddies paradox" whereby, in their studies, large-scale irrigation projects are themselves malaria neutral, selecting for less anthropophilic *Anopheles* mosquito spp., but appear to drive malaria in outlying regions, including highlands and desert fringes, whose populace host lesser herd immunity and have little access to bed nets and healthcare.

Chaves's group (2008) extends the descriptions of these processes to more explicitly connect the proximate social ecologies many researchers favor to the mechanisms of expropriation at the core of both plantation economies and neoliberal production:

> The association between outbreaks and forest clearance, higher risk for populations living close to forests, and the absence of [American Cutaneous Leishmaniasis, another vector-borne disease] from urban settings has led to the proposal that it will disappear with the destruction of primary forests. This view ignores the complex nature of deforestation as a product of socioeconomic inequities...

> Contrary to the established view, living close to the forest edge can diminish the risk provided other factors are taken into account. Additionally, differences in vulnerability to climatic variability appear to interact with forest cover to influence risk across counties where the disease has its largest burden. Incidence exacerbation associated with El Niño Southern Oscillation is observed in counties with larger proportions of deforestation.

Chaves et al. explicitly connect deforestation, commercial agriculture, and social marginalization to the sudden success of a vector-borne pathogen:

> The risk of infection is diminished among those living close to forests, an unexpected pattern in light of previous studies on the role of this habitat type. The pathway by which social marginalization promotes transmission of Leishmania in this context probably is linked to a major environmental problem affecting the tropics: destruction of forests and associated biodiversity.

> Forest clearing worldwide, and especially in Costa Rica, is concurrent with development of large scale commercial agriculture, including monocultures of several commercial crops where ACL is clustered, and with accelerated human population growth. This shift towards market-based agricultural production and rapidly expanding population is associated with new inequities in land tenure, increased numbers of landless peasants, and hence further pressure to cut down forests for local subsistence agriculture and extraction of other natural resources...

Clearly reversing deforestation is a necessary step in retaining ecosystemic services, biocontrol among them. But conservation is insufficient as both deforestation and reducing deforestation – the very green model millions support as Earth's salvation – are presently pursued on the neoliberal model of land expropriation and "efficient" agriculture intensification (Perfecto and Vandermeer 2010; Patel 2013). The forest embodies more than the number of trees conserved or lost. Preserving what the forest *does*, as opposed to what it *is*, must be grounded in a different episteme. A growing literature connects such matters of ownership and kinds of agricultural production to ecological outcome.

A meta-analysis by Gonthier et al. (2014) showed plant species richness increases with less intensive local management, while vertebrate richness increases with landscape complexity. Invertebrate richness responds to both. Chappell et al. (2013; Chappell 2018) found when supported by physical and human capital, with effective control of land transferred to peasants and governed in Ostrom-like common (Ostrom 1990; Allen et al. 2011), small-scale agroecological farming across complex land use mosaics in Brazil and elsewhere contributes to yields, farmer incomes, and conservation at local and landscape levels. A variety of ecosystem services are promoted, including wildlife diversity, agrobiodiversity, wildlife corridors, seed dispersal, pollination services, carbon sequestration, buffer zones, pollution control, and pest and disease control.

Along with price controls and subsidies, community resilience can be built-in as a landscape basic. A diversity of produce within and across farms, by *Milpa* polyculture in Mexico, for instance, means that food remains available even when production proves seasonally unprofitable.

4.2   Modeling Capital-Led Epidemiology

Can these insights be teamed with the model approaches presented here to help introduce new lines of disease study and intervention? Is there room for a social epizoology and what might it look like?

An immediate possibility is that stochasticity can be put to work. In a comprehensive review of stochastic models in epidemiology, Isham (2005) notes that:

> Models will often need to incorporate *intrinsic* stochasticity. Thus, not only is there the long-acknowledged need to incorporate uncertainty in parameter values – generally achieved via a numerical sensitivity analysis – but, more importantly, the fact that the size of a population of infected hosts or of infecting parasites within a single host is random and integer-valued has many important consequences.

Among them, population stochasticity can be deterministic in origin and effect (Lewontin and Levins 2007). Here we explored the role dominant embedding socioeconomic paradigms play in deterministically imposing stochastic structures defining epidemic and pandemic dynamics. In two or more dimensions, the same underlying model — here for a host and vector system — can be driven either to extinction or explosion by different patterns and amplitudes of environmental "noise."

Under one noise framework, mosaicking geographies and ecosystemic functions stabilize disease systems, while smoothing them out with economies of scale explosively destabilizes them. Diseconomies of scale of grave damage routinely accompany the latter. Simply the erosive removal of mosaicking in space, time, and/or agroecological mode, or, at the other geographical terminus, defunding urban environmental sanitation, can be sufficient to trigger an explosive pathogen outbreak. On the other hand, for dimensions two or greater, a structural shift to certain kinds of cross-influence noise will, after an amplitude threshold, drive explosive outbreaks. There are a number of possible mechanisms for the latter: by metapopulation rescue, synchronized bursts of vector population and host availability, a surge in characteristic area that shifts the system off its demographic floor or helps select for a better fit between host and vector, or a socioeconomic Moran effect that overlaps environmental noise for host and vector.

The details will be ecosystem-specific and may be counterintuitive. That is, what seems a "simple" or even "minor" adventure in agroecological exploitation or urban planning may prove to be neither in a complex ecosystem.

With Ross (1911) and his followers, public policy and its intertwinings with socioeconomic structure under the rubric of "public health" were discovered to determine the fundamental parameters of deterministic models of vector-borne diseases. One can, then, by proper vector control in a socioeconomically stable context, drive Zika, malaria, and other vector-borne pathogens to very low endemic levels, even to local extirpation.

Neoliberal and other kinds of exploitation can scramble long-selected patterns and processes associated with said protection even when "public health" measures are kept in place. That interference alone may suffice to trigger explosive outbreaks of even previously marginalized vector-borne infections or ratchets in public health degradation. In reality, of course, both the agroecological context defining mosquito dynamics and the public health programs ostensibly directed to countermand them suffer from ideologically driven structural adjustment. Zika will unlikely be the last "new infection" to germinate in the neoliberal plantations and periurbanized slums of the global south.

We should be able to better conceptually assimilate, and with the right political alignment even reverse, such trajectories. Economic-geographic markers of global capitalism's impacts upon agricultural landscapes (including the pathogens within) can be operationalized in terms of the ecosystem services lost or gained – environmental stochasticity's biocontrol among them. For instance, we might set such broadly painted political economies in absolute geographies that include hectares leased to multinationals per total agricultural area, the number of farms consolidated in the past decade, and the volatility of the prices of food commodities grown for multiple markets domestic and export.

On the other hand, agroeconomics and associated diseases are marked by relational geographies across industrial regions and sectors (Cummins et al. 2007; Bergmann 2013; Wallace et al. 2015, 2016; Bergmann and Holmberg 2016; Bergmann 2017). Landscapes are entrained by transnational commodity chains and circuits of capital, including financial and productive circuits, with critical local effects. Products from globalized croplands, forests, or pastures eventually contribute to consumption or capital accumulation in other countries. Other landscapes are enmeshed primarily within local circuits of production and exchange. Bergmann and Holmberg (2016) extend analysis beyond characterizing landscapes that directly produce traditional agricultural exports to identifying the forests and fields that are part of commodity webs supporting export-oriented development, producing goods or services for international markets. The team further differentiates foreign consumption/accumulation of "direct" agricultural goods, processed agricultural goods, manufactured goods as far afield as electronics and vehicles, and services, including air transport, insurance, and education. Bergmann (2013, 2017) extends these relational geographies to carbon emissions and labor intensity.

How these economic circuits structure disease ecologies – marketization, expansion of processing industries and infrastructure needed to scale up the market areas, and potential uses of given agriculture, increases in scale of parcel size and monocultural uniformity – is a matter of ongoing research. Such broad impact – as measured by way of the life cycle analyses, ecological footprinting, and input-output analyses of industrial ecology – might produce large-scale ecosystemic shifts that set off spikes in pathogen population or cladogenesis, inducing new patterns of transmission, virulence, and endemicity. That is, through specific commodities or bundles thereof, changes in policy or socioeconomic structure can trigger a large-scale biological logic gate that frees a pathogen that up to an outbreak had been held at a low endemic level (or had not previously evolved) (Wallace et al. 2016).

Higher-order shifts along global circuits of capital domestically interpenetrate land-use changes that disconnect (and reconnect) local epidemiologies across host species. Even if by capitalism's impacts those relationships have changed in scale and effect, disease, culture, ecology, and power have long interpenetrated each other. From civilization's origins, and multiple reinventions, such shifts have repeatedly selected for novel outbreaks, of which Zika and other novel and reemergent vector-borne pathogens appear on a growing list of recent examples (McNeill 1977/2010; Dobson and Carper 1996; Wolfe et al. 2007; FAO 2013; Engering et al. 2013; Wallace et al. 2015).

Contrast such a proposed program in research and intervention with cost-effectiveness analysis, much of which implicitly accepts the premises of a social system of extraordinary inequity whose operational directives facilitate the repeated emergence of vector-borne infections to begin with (e.g., Owen et al. 2012; Tozan et al. 2014; Golding et al. 2015; Shim 2016). Even as some such analyses favor massive expenditures in virus control to preclude, for instance, Zika's clear medical burden (Alfaro-Murillo et al. 2016), and others make the distinction between productive and allocative efficiencies (Segall 2003), the preponderance of such research organizes an ethics of economism around minimizing immediate expenditures for particular institutions first, rather than protecting communities or addressing the structural expropriation that produces the very artificial scarcities these analyses ostensibly address (Farmer 2008; Sparke 2009; Chiriboga et al. 2015; Sparke 2017).

Other modeling frameworks arrive at similarly problematic conclusions. Coleman et al. (2001) appropriate the agricultural concept of endemic stability for a broader range of diseases. The stability is defined as a population state in which clinical disease is rare even as the level of infection is high. In some parts of such a disease parameter space, partial intervention, retarding the force of infection, can exacerbate disease incidence by weakening herd immunity. Sometimes doing nothing may be the best intervention. Some groups have proposed just letting Zika, which causes little clinical expression in most cases, burn out as the best approach (Ferrara 2016).

While clearly the ecological damage in eliminating mosquito spp. need be avoided – from indiscriminate pesticide application to disruptions in food webs – the epidemic of poverty-associated microcephaly and the reciprocal activation Zika shares with dengue make "doing nothing" here unconscionable. Austerity programs – and transgenic fixes – are by no means the only way to circumvent the environmental damage associated with pesticide-led interventions. Community- and region-level interventions in housing, sanitation, and other social and ecological determinants of health specific to vector-borne infection can have profound impact, including eliminating disease (David et al. 2007; Taylor 2009; Arunachalam et al. 2010; Bermudez-Tamayo et al. 2016; Costa et al. 2017; Xu et al. 2017). Another science has long been possible.

Epistemologies, even deep into their mathematical formalisms, however useful they may be, are political in nature (Levins 1998, 2006; Winther 2006; Wallace 2011; Schizas 2012; Nikisianis and Stamou 2016). Control theory as deployed here, for instance, represents an anti-neoliberal model of intervention if only because it assumes state intervention in favor of the commons. In this case, it presumes a public good in preserving the veritably free stochastic ecosystemic services even human-integrated forests provide and that fairly cheap public health and sanitation services can impose upon cities, short-circuiting disease transmission *before* an outbreak. Capital, in contrast, treats nature as a competitor over the right to supply ecosystemic services and appears maneuvering to turn more than just now-bottled water into fictitious commodities (Polanyi 1944/2001; Jaffee and Newman 2013; Wallace 2017). Agribusiness has already stripped out ecosystems to its financial advantage, more than just growing export crops, but also by commoditizing soil fertility and pest control into inputs for which farmers must turn over nearly the totality of their revenue (Wallace 2016a, b; Qualman 2017; Chappell 2018). One need not oppose pharmaceuticals and other prophylaxes as a class to see such efforts appear now to extend to the means by which to address the very pandemics the food sector helps generate.

Mirowski (2009, 2015) framed such machination in decidedly stark terms, with foundational implications for the practice of science:

> *The market (suitably reengineered and promoted) can always provide solutions to problems seemingly caused by the market in the first place.* This is the ultimate destination of the constructivist orientation within neoliberalism. Any problem, economic or otherwise, has a market solution, given sufficient ingenuity: pollution is abated by the trading of emissions permits; inadequate public education is rectified by vouchers; auctions can adequately structure communication channels... Poverty-striken sick people lacking access to healthcare can be incentivized to serve as guinea pigs for clinical drug trials... Because the marketplace is deemed to be a superior information processor, all human knowledge can only be used to its fullest if it is comprehensively owned and priced.

Pathogens, fast-evolving, some threatening billions outside expedient models of risk, routinely refuse to cooperate with such a lucrative metaphysics, infecting people who cannot pay market rates with diseases the market cannot cure.

References

Alfaro-Murillo, J. A., Parpia, A. S., Fitzpatrick, M. C., Tamagnan, J. A., Medlock, J., Ndeffo-Mbah, M.L., Fish, D., Avila-Agero, M.L., Marin, R., Ko, A.I., Galvani, A.P., 2016, A cost-effectiveness tool for informing policies on Zika virus control, PLoS Negl Trop Dis., 10(5):e0004743.

Ali, S., Gugliemini, O., Harber, S., Harrison, A., Houle, L., et al., 2017, Environmental and social change drive the explosive emergence of Zika virus in the Americas, PLoS Neglected Tropical Diseases. doi: https://doi.org/10.1371/journal.pntd.0005135.

Allen, J., DuVander, J., Kubiszewski, I., Ostrom, E., 2011, Institutions for managing ecosystem services, Solutions, 2(6):44–48.

Amankwah, K., Klerkx, L., Sakyi-Dawson, O., Karbo, N., Oosting, S.J., Leeuwis, C., and van der Zijpp, A.J., 2014, Institutional dimensions of veterinary services reforms: responses to structural adjustment in Northern Ghana, International Journal of Agricultural Sustainability 12(3). Available online at https://doi.org/10.1080/14735903.2014.909635.

Arunachalam, N., Tana, S., Espino, F., Kittayapong, P., Abeyewickreme, W., Thet Wai, K., Kishore Tyagi, B., Kroeger, A., Sommerfeld, J., Petzold, M., 2010, Eco-bio-social determinants of dengue vector breeding: a multicountry study in urban and periurban Asia, Bull World Health Organ, 88:173184.

Bergmann, L.R., 2013, Bound by chains of carbon: Ecological-economic geographies of globalization, Annals of the Association of American Geographers, 103:13481370.

Bergmann, L.R., 2017, Towards economic geographies beyond the Nature-Society divide, Geoforum, 85:324–335.

Bergmann, L.R., Holmberg, M., 2016, Land in motion, Annals of the American Association of Geographers, 106(4):932–956.

Bermudez-Tamayo, C., Mukamana, O., Carabali, M., Osorio, L., Fournet, F., Dabir, K.R., Marteli, C.T., Contreras, A., Ridde, V., 2016, Priorities and needs for research on urban interventions targeting vector-borne diseases: rapid review of scoping and systematic reviews, Infectious Diseases of Poverty, 5:104. doi: https://doi.org/10.1186/s40249-016-0198-6.

Caprara, A., Lima, J.W., Marinho, A.C., Calvasina, P.G., Landim, L.P., Sommerfeld, J., 2009, Irregular water supply, household usage and dengue: a bio-social study in the Brazilian Northeast, Cad Saude Publica., 25 Suppl 1:S125–S136.

Carlson, C.J., Dougherty, E.R., Getz, W., 2016, An ecological assessment of the pandemic threat of Zika virus, PLoS Neglected Tropical Diseases, 10(8):e0004968.

Celli, A., 1900, Malaria According to the New Researches, Longmans, Green and Co, London.

Celli, A., 1925, Storia della Malaria nell'Agro Romano. Opera postuma con illustrazioni del Dott. P. Ambrogetti e una Carta Topografca, Mem. R. Accad. Linei, 1(6):73–467.

Chappell, M.J., 2018, Beginning to End Hunger: Food and the Environment in Belo Horizonte, Brazil, and Beyond, University of California Press, Berkeley.

Chappell, M.J., Wittman, H., Bacon, C.M., Ferguson, B.G., Barrios, L.G., Barrios, R.G., Jaffee, D., Lima, J., Méndez, V.E., Morales, H., Soto-Pinto, L., Vandermeer, J., Perfecto, I., 2013, Food sovereignty: an alternative paradigm for poverty reduction and biodiversity conservation in Latin America, F1000Res, 2:235.

Chaves, L.F., 2013, The dynamics of Latifundia formation, PLoS ONE, 8(12):e82863.

Chaves, L.F., Cohen, J.M., Pascual, M., Wilson, M.L., 2008, Social exclusion modifies climate and deforestation impacts on a vector-borne disease, PLoS Neglected Tropical Diseases, 2(2):e176. Available online at https://doi.org/10.1371/journal.pntd.0000176.

Chiriboga, D. Buss, P. Birn, A.E., Garay, J., Muntaner, C., Nervi, L., 2015, Investing in health, The Lancet, 383(9921):949.

Coleman, P.G., Perry, B.D., Woolhouse, M.E.J., 2001, Endemic stability a veterinary idea applied to human public health, The Lancet, 357(9264):12841286.

Costa, F., Carvalho-Pereira, T., Begon, M., Riley, L., Childs, J., 2017, Zoonotic and vector-borne diseases in urban slums: opportunities for intervention, Trends Parasitol., 33(9):660–662.

Cummins, S., Curtis, S., Diez-Roux, A.V., Macintyre, S., 2007, Understanding and representing 'place' in health research: A relational approach, Social Science & Medicine, 65:1825–1838.

David, A.M., Mercado, S.P., Becker, D., Edmundo, K., Mugisha, F., 2007, The prevention and control of HIV/AIDS, TB and vector-borne diseases in informal settlements: challenges, opportunities and insights. Journal of Urban Health, 84(S1):6574.

Dobson, A.P., Carper, E.R., 1996, Infectious diseases and human population history, BioScience, 46(2):126.

Dzingirai, V., Bukachi, S., Leach, M., Mangwanya, L., Scoones, I., and Wilkinson, A., 2017, Structural drivers of vulnerability to zoonotic disease in Africa. Phil. Trans. R. Soc. B, 372(1725):20160169.

Engering, A., Hogerwerf, L., Slingenbergh, J., 2013, Pathogen host environment interplay and disease emergence, Emerging Microbes and Infections, 2:e5.

Enticott, G., Donaldson, A., Lowe, P., Power, M., Proctor, A., and Wilkinson, K. (2011) The changing role of veterinary expertise in the food chain. Phil. Trans. R. Soc. B, 366:1955–1965.

FAO, 2013, World Livestock 2013: Changing Disease Landscapes, Food and Agriculture Organization, United Nations, Rome.

Farmer, P., 2008, Challenging orthodoxies: the road ahead for health and human rights, Health Hum. Rights, 10(1):519.

Ferrara, J., 2016, An easy solution to the war on Zika? Experts say eradicating mosquitoes is not the answer. ScienceLine, 9 May. Available online at http://scienceline.org/2016/05/an-easy-solution-to-the-war-on-zika/.

Foster, J.B., Clark, B., York, R., 2010, The Ecological Rift: Capitalism's War on the Earth, Monthly Review Press, New York.

Golding, N., Wilson, A.L., Moyes, C.L., Cano, J., Pigott, D.M., Velayudhan, R., Brooker, S.J., Smith, D.L., Hay, S.I., Lindsay, S.W., 2015, Integrating vector control across diseases, BMC Med., 13:249.

Gonthier, D.J., Ennis, K.K., Farinas, S., Hsieh, H.Y., Iverson, A.L., Batáry, P., Rudolphi, J., Tscharntke, T., Cardinale, B.J., Perfecto, I., 2014, Biodiversity conservation in agriculture requires a multi-scale approach, Proc Biol Sci., 281(1791):20141358.

Ijumba, J.N., Lindsay, S.W., 2001, Impact of irrigation on malaria in Africa: paddies paradox, Med Vet Entomol., 15(1):1–11.

Isham, V., 2005, Stochastic Models for Epidemics, Chapter 1 in Davison, A., Y. Dodge, W. Wermuth (eds.), Celebrating Statistics: Papers in Honour of Sir David Cox on his 80th Birthday, Oxford University Press, London.

Jaffee, D., Newman, S., 2013, A more perfect commodity: Bottled water, global accumulation, and local contestation, Rural Sociology, 78(1):1–28.

Johnson, C. 2017, Pregnant woman versus mosquito: A feminist epidemiology of Zika virus, Journal of International Political Theory, 13(2):233250.

Jones, B.A., Betson, M., Pfeiffer, D.U., 2017, Eco-social processes influencing infectious disease emergence and spread, Parasitology, 144(1):26–36.

Kelly, A.H., Lezaun, J., 2014, Urban mosquitoes, situational publics, and the pursuit of interspecies separation in Dar es Salaam, American Ethnologist, 41(2):368–383.

Kentikelenis, A., Karanikolos, M., Aaron Reeves, A., Martin McKee, M., Stuckler, D., 2014, Greece's health crisis: from austerity to denialism, The Lancet, 383(9918):748–753.

Levins, R., 1998, The internal and external in explanatory theories, Science as Culture, 7(4):557–582.

Levins, R., 2006, Strategies of abstraction, Biol Philos, 21:741–755.

Lewontin, R., Levins, R., 2007, Chance and necessity. In Biology Under the Influence: Dialectical Essays on Ecology, Agriculture, and Health. Monthly Review Press, New York.

Lindsay, S., Emerson, P.M., Charlwood, J.D., 2002, Reducing malaria by mosquito-proofing houses, Trends in Parasitology, 18(11):510–514.

McNeill, W.H., 1977/2010, Plagues and Peoples, Knopf Doubleday Publishing Group, New York.

Mirowski, P., 2009, Postface: defining neoliberalism, In P. Mirowski, D. Plehwe (eds), The Road From Mont Pélerin: The Making of the Neoliberal Thought Collective, Harvard University Press, Cambridge.

Mirowski, P., 2015, Science-Mart: Privatizing American Science, Havard University Press, Cambridge.

Mota, M.T., Terzian, A.C., Silva, M.L., Estofolete, C., Nogueira, M.L., 2016, Mosquito-transmitted viruses - the great Brazilian challenge, Braz J Microbiol., 47 Suppl 1:38–50.

Moore, J.W., 2015, Capitalism in the Web of Life: Ecology and the Accumulation of Capital, Verso, New York.

Muntaner, C., Wallace, R.G., 2018. Confronting the social and environmental determinants of health. In H. Waitzkin (ed), Health Care Under the Knife: Moving Beyond Capitalism for Our Health, Monthly Review Press, New York.

Nading, A.M., 2014, Mosquito Trails: Ecology, Health, and the Politics of Entanglement, University of California Press, Berkeley.

Nikisianis, N., Stamou, G.P., 2016, Harmony as ideology: Questioning the diversity- stability hypothesis, Acta Biotheoretica, 64(1):33–64.

Ostrom, E., 1990, Governing the Commons: The Evolution of Institutions for Collective Action, Cambridge University Press, Cambridge.

Owen, L., Morgan, A., Fischer, A., Ellis, S., Hoy, A., Kelly, M.P., 2012, The cost-effectiveness of public health interventions, J Public Health, 34(1):37–45.

Patel, R., 2013, The Long Green Revolution, The Journal of Peasant Studies, 40(1):1–63.

Perfecto, I., Vandermeer, J., 2010, The agroecological matrix as alternative to the land-sparing/agriculture intensification model, Proc Natl Acad Sci U S A, 107(13):57865791.

Pfeiffer, J., Chapman, R., 2010, Anthropological perspectives on structural adjustment and public health, Annu. Rev. Anthropol., 39:149–165.

Polanyi, K., 1944/2001, The Great Transformation: The Political and Economic Origins of Our Time, Beacon Press, Boston.

Qualman, D., 2017, Agribusiness takes all: 90 years of Canadian net farm income, Darrin Qualman blog, February 28. Available online at http://www.darrinqualman.com/canadian-net-farm-income/.

Ross, R., 1911, The Prevention of Malaria, Second Edition, Murray, London.

Schizas, D., 2012, Systems ecology reloaded: A critical assessment focusing on the relations between science and ideology. In G.P. Stamou (ed), Populations, Biocommunities, Ecosystems: A Review of Controversies in Ecological Thinking. Bentham Science Publishers, Sharjah.

Segall, M., 2003, District health systems in a neoliberal world: a review of five key policy areas, Int J Health Plann Mgmt, 18:S5–S26.

Shim, E., 2016, Dengue dynamics and vaccine cost-effectiveness analysis in the Philippines, Am J Trop Med Hyg., 95(5):1137–1147.

Shragai, T., Tesla, B., Murdock, C., Harrington, L.C., 2017, Zika and chikungunya: mosquito-borne viruses in a changing world, Annals of the New York Academy of Science, 1399(1):61–77.

Sparke, M., 2009, Unpacking economism and remapping the terrain of global health, In A. Kay, O.D. Williams (eds), Global Health Governance: Crisis, Institutions and Political Economy, Springer, Switzerland.

Sparke, M., 2016, Health and the embodiment of neoliberalism: Pathologies of political economy from climate change and austerity to personal responsibility. In S. Springer, K. Birch, and J. MacLeavy (eds), Handbook of Neoliberalism, Routledge, New York.

Sparke, M., 2017, Austerity and the embodiment of neoliberalism as ill-health: Towards a theory of biological sub-citizenship, Social Science Medicine, 187:287–295.

Tabachnick, W.J., 2016, Ecological effects on arbovirus-mosquito cycles of transmission, Current Opinion in Virology, 21:124–131.

Taylor, S., 2009, Political epidemiology: strengthening socio-political analysis for mass immunisation - lessons from the smallpox and polio programmes, Glob Public Health, 4(6):546–560.

Tozan, Y., Ratanawong, P., Louis, V.R., Kittayapong, P., Wilder-Smith, A., 2014, Use of insecticide-treated school uniforms for prevention of dengue in schoolchildren: a cost-effectiveness analysis, PLoS One, 9(9):e108017.

Vittor, A., 2016, Explainer: where did Zika virus come from and why is it a problem in Brazil? The Conversation, 27 January. Available online at https://theconversation.com/explainer-where-did-zika-virus-come-from-and-why-is-it-a-problem-in-brazil-53425.

Vittor, A., Gilman, R., Tielsch, J., Glass, G., Shields, T., Sanchez-Lozano, W., Pinedo-Cancino, V., Patz, J., 2006, The effects of deforestation on the human-biting rate of *Anopheles darlingi*, the primary vector of Falciparium Malaria in the Peruvian Amazon, American Journal of Tropical Medicine and Hugiene, 74:3–11.

Vittor, A., Gilman, R., Tielsch, J., Glass, G., Shields, T., Sanchez- Lozano, W., Pinedo, V., et al., 2009, Linking deforestation to Malaria in the Amazon: Characterization of the breeding habitat of the principal Malaria vector *Anopheles darlingi*, American Journal of Torpical Medicine and Hygiend, 81:5–12.

Wallace, R., Bergmann, L., Hogerwerf, L., Kock, R., Wallace, R.G., 2016, Ebola in the hog sector: Modeling pandemic emergence in commodity livestock, In R.G. Wallace and R. Wallace (eds.), Neoliberal Ebola: Modeling Disease Emergence from Finance to Forest and Farm. Springer, Switzerland.

Wallace, R.G., 2011, Occupy mathematics, Farming Pathogens blog, November 8. Available online at https://farmingpathogens.wordpress.com/2011/11/08/occupy-mathematics/.

Wallace, R.G., 2016a, Big Farms Make Big Flu: Dispatches on Infectious Disease, Agribusiness, and the Nature of Science. Monthly Review Press, New York.

Wallace, R.G., 2016b, Strange cotton, In Big Farms Make Big Flu: Dispatches on Infectious Diseases, Agribusiness, and the Nature of Science, Monthly Review Press, New York.

Wallace, R.G., 2017. Impermissible exchange. Farming Pathogens blog, July 11. Available online at https://farmingpathogens.wordpress.com/2017/07/11/impermissible-exchange/.

Wallace, R.G., Alders, R., Kock, R., Jonas, T., Wallace, R., Hogerwerf, L., 2018, Health before medicine: Community resilience in food landscapes, In M. Walton (ed.), One Planet - Eco-One Health: Looking After Humans, Animals and the Environment, Sydney University Press, Sydney.

Wallace, R.G., Bergmann, L., Kock, R., Gilbert, M., Hogerwerf, L., Wallace, R., Holmberg, M., 2015, The dawn of Structural One Health: A new science tracking disease emergence along circuits of capital, Social Science and Medicine, 129:68–77.

Weaver, S.C., Reisen, W.K., 2010, Present and future arboviral threats, Antiviral Res., 85(2):328.

Weber, D.S., Alroy, K.A., Scheiner, S.M., 2017, Phylogenetic insight into Zika and emerging viruses for a perspective on potential hosts, Ecohealth, 14(2):214–218.

Winther, R.G., 2006, On the dangers of making scientific models ontologically independent: taking Richard Levins' warnings seriously, Biol Philos, 21:703–724.

Wolfe, N. D., Dunavan, C. P., Diamond, J., 2007, Origins of major human infectious diseases, Nature, 447:279283.

Xu, J.W., Li, J.J., Guo, H.P., Pu, S.W., Li, S.M., Wang, R.H., Liu, H., Wang, W.J., 2017, Malaria from hyperendemicity to elimination in Hekou County on China-Vietnam border: an ecological study, Malar J., 16(1):66. doi: https://doi.org/10.1186/s12936-017-1709-z.

Chapter 5
Mathematical Appendix

5.1 Morse Theory

Morse theory examines relations between analytic behavior of a function – the location and character of its critical points – and the underlying topology of the manifold on which the function is defined. We are interested in a number of such functions, for example, information source uncertainty on a parameter space and "second-order" iterations involving parameter manifolds determining critical behavior, among them the sudden onset of a giant component in a network model. To present some of the basics here, we follow Pettini (2007).

The central argument of Morse theory is to examine an n-dimensional manifold M as decomposed into level sets of some function $f: M \to \mathbf{R}$ where $\mathbf{R}$ is the set of real numbers. The a-level set of f is defined as

$$f^{-1}(a) = \{x \in M : f(x) = a\},$$

the set of all points in M with $f(x) = a$. If M is compact, then the whole manifold can be decomposed into such slices in a canonical fashion between two limits, defined by the minimum and maximum of f on M. Let the part of M below a be defined as

$$M_a = f^{-1}(-\infty, a] = \{x \in M : f(x) \le a\}.$$

These sets describe the whole manifold as a varies between the minimum and maximum of f.

Morse functions are defined as a particular set of smooth functions $f: M \to \mathbf{R}$ as follows. Suppose a function f has a critical point x_c, so that the derivative $df(x_c) = 0$,

© Springer International Publishing AG 2018
R. Wallace et al., *Clear-Cutting Disease Control*,
https://doi.org/10.1007/978-3-319-72850-6_5

with critical value $f(x_c)$. Then f is a Morse function if its critical points are nondegenerate in the sense that the Hessian matrix J of second derivatives at x_c, whose elements, in terms of local coordinates, are

$$J_{i,j} = \partial^2 f / \partial x^i \partial x^j,$$

has rank n, which means that it has only nonzero eigenvalues, so that there are no lines or surfaces of critical points and, ultimately, critical points are isolated.

The index of the critical point is the number of negative eigenvalues of J at x_c. A level set $f^{-1}(a)$ of f is called a critical level if a is a critical value of f, that is, if there is at least one critical point $x_c \in f^{-1}(a)$.

Again following Pettini (2007), the essential results of Morse theory are as follows:

1. If an interval $[a, b]$ contains no critical values of f, then the topology of $f^{-1}[a, v]$ does not change for any $v \in (a, b]$. Importantly, the result is valid even if f is not a Morse function, but only a smooth function.
2. If the interval $[a, b]$ contains critical values, the topology of $f^{-1}[a, v]$ changes in a manner determined by the properties of the matrix J at the critical points.
3. If $f: M \rightarrow \mathbf{R}$ is a Morse function, the set of all the critical points of f is a discrete subset of M, i.e., critical points are isolated. This is Sard's theorem.
4. If $f: M \rightarrow \mathbf{R}$ is a Morse function, with M compact, then on a finite interval $[a, b] \subset \mathbf{R}$, there is only a finite number of critical points p of f such that $f(p) \in [a, b]$. The set of critical values of f is a discrete set of $\mathbf{R}$.
5. For any differentiable manifold M, the set of Morse functions on M is an open dense set in the set of real functions of M of differentiability class r for $0 \leq r \leq \infty$.
6. Some topological invariants of M, that is, quantities that are the same for all the manifolds that have the same topology as M, can be estimated and sometimes computed exactly once all the critical points of f are known: let the Morse numbers $\mu_i (i = 0, ..., m)$ of a function f on M be the number of critical points of f of index i, (the number of negative eigenvalues of H). The Euler characteristic of the complicated manifold M can be expressed as the alternating sum of the Morse numbers of any Morse function on M,

$$X = \sum_{i=1}^{m} (-1)^i \mu_i.$$

The Euler characteristic reduces, in the case of a simple polyhedron, to

$$X = V - E + F$$

where V, E, and F are the numbers of vertices, edges, and faces in the polyhedron.

7. Another important theorem states that if the interval $[a, b]$ contains a critical value of f with a single critical point x_c, then the topology of the set M_b defined above differs from that of M_a in a way which is determined by the index, i, of the

critical point. Then M_b is homeomorphic to the manifold obtained from attaching to M_a an i-handle, i.e., the direct product of an i-disk and an $(m - i)$-disk.

Matsumoto (2002) and Pettini (2007) provide details and further references.

5.2 Groupoids

Given a pairing, for example, a connection by a meaningful path to the same base-point, it is possible to define "natural" end-point maps $\alpha(g) = a_j$, $\beta(g) = a_k$ from the set of morphisms G into A, and a formally associative product in the groupoid $g_1 g_2$ provided $\alpha(g_1 g_2) = \alpha(g_1)$, $\beta(g_1 g_2) = \beta(g_2)$, and $\beta(g_1) = \alpha(g_2)$. Then the product is defined, and associative, i.e., $(g_1 g_2) g_3 = g_1 (g_2 g_3)$, with the inverse defined by $g = (a_j, a_k)$, $g^{-1} \equiv (a_k, a_j)$.

In addition there are natural left and right identity elements λ_g, ρ_g such that $\lambda_g g = g = g \rho_g$.

An orbit of the groupoid G over A is an equivalence class for the relation $a j \sim G a_k$ if and only if there is a groupoid element g with $\alpha(g) = a_j$ and $\beta(g) = a_k$. Following Cannas Da Silva and Weinstein (1999), a groupoid is called transitive if it has just one orbit. The transitive groupoids are the building blocks of groupoids in that there is a natural decomposition of the base space of a general groupoid into orbits. Over each orbit there is a transitive groupoid, and the disjoint union of these transitive groupoids is the original groupoid. Conversely, the disjoint union of groupoids is itself a groupoid.

The isotropy group of $a \in X$ consists of those g in G with $\alpha(g) = a = \beta(g)$. These groups prove fundamental to classifying groupoids.

If G is any groupoid over A, the map (α, β): $G \to A \times A$ is a morphism from G to the pair groupoid of A. The image of (α, β) is the orbit equivalence relation $\sim G$, and the functional kernel is the union of the isotropy groups. If f: $X \to Y$ is a function, then the kernel of f, $ker(f) = [(x_1, x_2) \in X \times X: f(x_1) = f(x_2)]$ defines an equivalence relation.

Groupoids may have additional structure. As Weinstein (1996) explains, a groupoid G is a topological groupoid over a base space X if G and X are topological spaces and α, β and multiplication are continuous maps. A criticism sometimes applied to groupoid theory is that their classification up to isomorphism is nothing other than the classification of equivalence relations via the orbit equivalence relation and groups via the isotropy groups. The imposition of a compatible topological structure produces a nontrivial interaction between the two structures. Below we will introduce a metric structure on manifolds of related information sources, producing such interaction.

In essence a groupoid is a category in which all morphisms have an inverse, here defined in terms of connection by a meaningful path of an information source dual to a cognitive process.

As Weinstein (1996) points out, the morphism (α, β) suggests another way of looking at groupoids. A groupoid over A identifies not only which elements of A are equivalent to one another (isomorphic), but *it also parameterizes the different ways (isomorphisms) in which two elements can be equivalent*, i.e., all possible information sources dual to some cognitive process. Given the information theoretic characterization of cognition presented above, this produces a full modular cognitive network in a highly natural manner.

Brown (1987) describes the basic structure as follows:

A groupoid should be thought of as a group with many objects, or with many identities. A groupoid with one object is essentially just a group. So the notion of groupoid is an extension of that of groups. It gives an additional convenience, flexibility and range of applications...

EXAMPLE 1. A disjoint union [of groups] $G = \cup_\lambda G_\lambda$, $\lambda \in \Lambda$, is a groupoid: the product ab is defined if and only if a, b belong to the same G_λ and ab is then just the product in the group G_λ. There is an identity 1_λ for each $\lambda \in \Lambda$. The maps α, β coincide and map G_λ to λ, $\lambda \in \Lambda$.

EXAMPLE 2. An equivalence relation R on [a set] X becomes a groupoid with α, β: $R \rightarrow X$ the two projections, and product $(x, y)(y, z) = (x, z)$ whenever (x, y), $(y, z) \in R$. There is an identity, namely (x, x), for each $x \in X$ ...

Weinstein (1996) makes the following fundamental point:

Almost every interesting equivalence relation on a space B arises in a natural way as the orbit equivalence relation of some groupoid G over B. Instead of dealing directly with the orbit space B/G as an object in the category S_{map} of sets and mappings, one should consider instead the groupoid G itself as an object in the category $G_{ht\,p}$ of groupoids and homotopy classes of morphisms.

It is possible to explore homotopy in paths generated by information sources.

5.2.1   Global and Local Groupoids

The argument next follows Weinstein (1996) fairly closely, using his example of a finite tiling.

Consider a tiling of the euclidean plane R^2 by identical 2 by 1 rectangles, specified by the set X (one dimensional) where the grout between tiles is $X = H \cup V$, having $H = R \times Z$ and $V = 2Z \times R$, where R is the set of real numbers and Z the integers. Call each connected component of $R^2 \backslash X$, i.e., the complement of the two-dimensional real plane intersecting X, a tile.

Let Γ be the group of those rigid motions of R^2 which leave X invariant, i.e., the normal subgroup of translations by elements of the lattice $\Lambda = H \cap V = 2Z \times Z$ (corresponding to corner points of the tiles), together with reflections through each of the points $1/2\Lambda = Z \times 1/2Z$, and across the horizontal and vertical lines through those points. As noted in Weinstein (1996), much is lost in this coarse graining; in particular the same symmetry group would arise if we replaced X entirely by the lattice Λ of corner points. Γ retains no information about the local structure of the tiled plane. In the case of a real tiling, restricted to the finite set $B = [0, 2\,m] \times [0, n]$, the symmetry group shrinks drastically: The subgroup leaving $X \cap B$ invariant contains just four elements even though a repetitive pattern is clearly visible. A two-stage groupoid approach recovers the lost structure.

We define the transformation groupoid of the action of Γ on R^2 to be the set

$$G\left(\Gamma, R^2\right) = \{(x, \gamma, y | x \in R^2, y \in R^2, \gamma \in \Gamma, x = \gamma y\}$$

with the partially defined binary operation

$$(x, \gamma, y)(y, v, z) = (x, \gamma v, z).$$

Here $\alpha(x, \gamma, y) = x$, and $\beta(x, \gamma, y) = y$, and the inverses are natural.

We can form the restriction of G to B (or any other subset of R^2) by defining

$$G\left(\Gamma, R^2\right)\Big|_B = \left\{ g \in G\left(\Gamma, R^2\right) | \alpha(g), \beta(g) \in B \right\}$$

1. An orbit of the groupoid G over B is an equivalence class for the relation $x \sim G$ y if and only if there is a groupoid element g with $\alpha(g) = x$ and $\beta(g) = y$. Two points are in the same orbit if they are similarly placed within their tiles or within the grout pattern.
2. The isotropy group of $x \in B$ consists of those g in G with $\alpha(g) = x = \beta(g)$. It is trivial for every point except those in $1/2\Lambda \cap B$, for which it is $Z_2 \times Z_2$, i.e., the direct product of integers modulo two with itself.

By contrast, embedding the tiled structure within a larger context permits definition of a much richer structure, i.e., the identification of local symmetries.

We construct a second groupoid as follows: Consider the plane R^2 as being decomposed as the disjoint union of $P_1 = B \cap X$ (the grout), $P_2 = B \backslash P_1$ (the complement of P_1 in B, i.e., the tiles), and $P_3 = R_2 \backslash B$ (the exterior of the tiled room). Let E be the group of all euclidean motions of the plane, and define the local symmetry groupoid G_{loc} as the set of triples (x, γ, y) in $B \times E \times B$ for which $x = \gamma y$ and for which y has a neighborhood U in R^2 such that $\gamma(U \cap P_i) \subseteq P_i$ for $i = 1, 2, 3$. The composition is given by the same formula as for $G(\Gamma, R^2)$.

For this groupoid in context, there are only a finite number of orbits:

$O_1 =$ interior points of the tiles.
$O_2 =$ interior edges of the tiles.
$O_3 =$ interior crossing points of the grout.
$O_4 =$ exterior boundary edge points of the tile grout.
$O_5 =$ boundary "T" points.
$O_6 =$ boundary corner points.

The isotropy group structure is, however, now very rich indeed:

The isotropy group of a point in O_1 is now isomorphic to the entire rotation group O_2.
It is $Z_2 \times Z_2$ for O_2.
For O_3 it is the eight-element dihedral group D_4.
For O_4, O_5, and O_6, it is simply Z_2.
These are the "local symmetries" of the tile in context.

References

Brown, R., 1987, From groups to groupoids: a brief survey, Bulletin of the London Mathematical Society, 19:113–134.

Cannas Da Silva, A., Weinstein, A., 1999, Geometric Models for Noncommutative Algebras, American Mathematical Society, Providence, RI.

Matsumoto, Y., 2002, An Introduction to Morse Theory, American Mathematical Society, Provedence, RI.

Pettini, M., 2007, Geometry and Topology in Hamiltonian Dynamics, Springer, New York.

Weinstein, A., 1996, Groupoids: unifying internal and external symmetry, Notices of the American Mathematical Association, 43:744–752.

Printed in the United States
By Bookmasters